'Georgia's book is a must-read. She covers the subject matter with depth and credibility. Her writing style is accessible and inviting.'

— *Editor,* YOGA Magazine

'This is a lovely, thoughtful and accessible book incorporating shorter guided meditations for the start of class, meditations with hasta mudra, longer more detailed guided meditations and advice on how to create your own. It will provide a useful addition to the toolkit for yoga teachers and trainees. In the author's own words: "offering your students a little pocket of peace".'

— *Sian O'Neill, Editor of* Yoga Teaching Handbook *and* Yoga Student Handbook

'It is always a great joy to see past students create platforms for sharing the eternal wisdom of yoga with the community and I am delighted to endorse this fantastic piece of work by Georgia Keal. She has managed to make the ineffable teachings of classical yoga practical and relevant.

Georgia goes to great pains to establish the right setting and gives clear guidelines on how to prepare the space and create the right atmosphere so that it can easily become a part of your everyday life. She gives further guidance on how to sit or lie, how to use the breath and how to cultivate interoception (awareness of the body from within). The section on hand gestures (hasta mudras) is simple and easy to follow and the guided visualisations are well thought out. I will certainly be using ideas from this book myself and I hope you will too.'

— *Tarik Dervish, BWY Yoga Teacher/Trainer, Ayurvedic Practitioner*

T0271729

The Guided Meditation Handbook

of related interest

Yoga Teaching Handbook
A Practical Guide for Yoga Teachers and Trainees
Edited by Sian O'Neill
ISBN 978 1 84819 355 0
eISBN 978 0 85701 313 2

Ocean of Yoga
Meditations on Yoga and Ayurveda for Balance, Awareness and Well-Being
Julie Dunlop
Foreword by Vasant Lad, B.A.M. & S., M.A.Sc.
ISBN 978 1 84819 360 4
eISBN 978 0 85701 318 7

The Meditation Book of Light and Colour
Pauline Wills
ISBN 978 1 84819 202 7
eISBN 978 0 85701 162 6

Body Intelligence Meditation
Finding Presence through Embodiment
Ged Sumner
ISBN 978 1 84819 174 7
eISBN 978 0 85701 121 3

The Guided Meditation Handbook

Advice, Meditation Scripts
and Hasta Mudra for
Yoga Teachers

GEORGIA KEAL

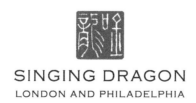

SINGING DRAGON
LONDON AND PHILADELPHIA

First published in 2020
by Singing Dragon
an imprint of Jessica Kingsley Publishers
73 Collier Street
London N1 9BE, UK
and
400 Market Street, Suite 400
Philadelphia, PA 19106, USA

www.singingdragon.com

Library of Congress Cataloging in Publication Data
A CIP catalog record for this book is available from the Library of Congress

British Library Cataloguing in Publication Data
A CIP catalogue record for this book is available from the British Library

ISBN 978 1 78775 048 7
eISBN 978 1 78775 049 4

Printed and bound by CPI Group (UK) Ltd, Croydon, CR0 4YY

Contents

Acknowledgements

I would like to thank Sarah Hamlin at Jessica Kingsley Publishers for all her time, support and helpful input throughout the creation of this book. Also thanks to Maddy Budd and Emma Holak at Jessica Kingsley Publishers. Thanks to my teacher Tarik Dervish for sharing his vast breadth of Yogic knowledge with myself and my fellow pupils throughout our BWY teacher training course and his continued support, including his helpful suggestions for this book. Thanks to the multi-talented photographer and yoga teacher Sarah Alice Lee for capturing the beautiful cover image, which was taken at the studio I teach at in Forest Row, Yard Yoga, and features the owner Sarah Campbell-Lloyd. Thanks to Sarah and her sister Daphne Harman-Clarke, owners of Yard Yoga, for being amazing, supportive and inspiring women. Thanks to all the wonderful teachers at Yard Yoga who nourish my body and inspire my practice with their wonderful lessons. Thanks to Sian O'Neill for her belief in this book from the very start. Thanks to my mum Carole Noddings for her boundless love, support and for introducing me to guided meditation. I have used her 'Blue Liquid' meditation since I was a child. Lastly, but by no means least, thanks to my husband Matt Keal, for his unwavering support, love, encouragement and countless cups of tea.

If you have any feedback on the book or if you would like to get in touch please email me at georgiakeal@hotmail.com

Introduction

How to use this book

This book is intended as a guide for yoga teachers, from trainees and beginners through to advanced practitioners, to enable them to share the positive benefits of guided meditation with their students. Although this handbook is primarily written for yoga teachers to use guided meditations in the setting of a yoga class, the contents and scripts of this book may also be useful for other types of practitioners who would like their students or clients to access the benefits of guided meditation.

Chapter 1 deals with all the aspects you need to consider when delivering a guided meditation in a yoga class, from the setting, to modifications, and everything in between. Chapter 2 covers short guided meditations to use at the beginning of the class with six scripts. These are designed to let the student switch off from their day and mentally arrive for the class. Chapter 3 covers *hasta mudras* with six meditation scripts, each exploring the benefits of different *hasta mudras*. Chapter 4 has six meditation scripts to be used at the end of the class. These scripts are slightly longer and explore different ways to cultivate a positive experience for the student. Chapter 5 outlines ways for you, the reader, to write your own scripts to deliver in your own class.

CHAPTER 1

Introduction to Guided Meditation

Benefits and Setting the Scene for Your Yoga Class

What is guided meditation and why is it needed in our modern world?

Guided meditation is when one person, the speaker, vocally guides another person or group of people into a deep state of relaxation. This generally begins with the students finding a comfortable position, either seated or lying down. The speaker will then guide the students into a relaxed state. This can be done in a number of ways, with the speaker focusing on the breath, bodily sensations or guided imagery.

The speaker may then offer some positive mental imagery or a guided story to further deepen the positive experience of the practice. When the mind is very relaxed it is receptive, and this can be used to improve a person's physical or mental wellbeing. The idea that the mind can influence the body has been used in therapeutic fields including psychology, medicine, neurobiology, science, religion and popular culture. It is essentially a placebo. No physical substance has entered the body, yet quantifiable positive results can be experienced after a guided meditation, and this 'placebo effect' has been used for centuries (Shapiro 1959). As the Buddha quoted, 'The mind is everything. What you think you become.' Therefore, any number of positive mental and physical states can be reached depending on the theme of the guided meditation. The speaker may use imagery or a story to release negative emotions or use the same techniques to cultivate positive ones. The speaker may paint a mental picture of a beautiful garden to further relax the students or take them on a journey to see their future selves to help them plan for a positive future. The possibilities are endless. The aim of a guided meditation is for the student to experience a noticeable improvement in their physical or mental wellbeing as a result of the practice.

Guided meditation is used in a number of settings – from yoga classes, to offices (Melville *et al.* 2012), to the treatment of post-traumatic stress disorder (PTSD) for soldiers (Jain *et al.* 2012), and its popularity and need is growing. It is used in mindfulness courses, Cognitive Behavioural Therapy (CBT) and, more recently, as online apps. The guided meditation app 'Calm' was downloaded more than 27 million times in 2017, and was named App of the Year by Apple, showing the growing popularity for guided meditation. Its founder, Michael Acton Smith, sees guided meditation becoming more widely used to balance our fast-paced lives, and believes it will rival jogging as an everyday exercise, but for the mind rather than the body.

In recent times, people are beginning to value strengthening the mind as much as they strengthen their bodies, to attain true wellbeing. People are realising the benefits of prioritising their 'mental immunity' in the same way they would look after their physical immunity by eating five portions of fruit and vegetables a day or by taking part in regular exercise. By making lifestyle choices and taking part in activities like these we can keep our bodies strong and healthy and are less susceptible to picking up physical illnesses. Mental immunity is a similar idea but applies to keeping our minds healthy and strong. Therefore, if we build up our mental immunity by learning techniques to help us cope with the stressors in our lives, we will be less susceptible to mental illnesses. Just like we work out our bodies, we should regularly give our minds a work-out to build those mental muscles. Taking ourselves from a stressed state to a relaxed state, more regularly, is one way to improve our mental immunity and the more we do this, the easier it will become. Stress can have so many negative effects on our physical and mental states

(Tosevski *et al.* 2006; Vyas *et al.* 2002), and meditation is a proven technique to effectively reduce stress (Goyal *et al.* 2014). As I explain below, guided meditation is the most accessible form of meditation, and a true tonic for the age we live in.

Benefits of guided meditation
Accessible

Some people may find it challenging to meditate, particularly at the beginning of cultivating a regular meditation practice. The mind has a natural tendency to wander, and we can lose the practice before we are able to experience the positive benefits of a meditation session. One of the main benefits of guided meditation is simply that it is guided. It doesn't matter if the mind wanders because the speaker is able to gently guide the listener back to the practice, allowing anyone to access the mindful, peaceful state that meditation offers.

Healing body and mind

Guided meditation can be used as a tool to heal the body and mind as it harnesses the positive effects of meditation and the power of visualisation. This powerful combination of guided imagery (visualisation) and meditation is a well-known technique in medical and scientific fields to bring about positive change in the treatment of patients (Elomaa, de Williams and Kalso 2009; Fernros, Furhoff and Wandell 2008; Wells 2010). The transformation can be surprisingly powerful and has been used in a number of settings. In a study using guided meditation in women with breast cancer, the practice led to incredible improvements including improved immune system functioning and increased natural cancer killer cells (Eremin *et al.* 2009). This shows that if the mind believes, the body responds and heals. Similarly, in a study that used guided meditation to treat soldiers who returned from active service with PTSD, guided meditation not only reduced symptoms of PTSD but also significantly improved their mental quality of life.

Additionally, the practice resulted in preventing PTSD and related symptoms from returning, making guided meditation a powerful tool in the positive transformation of the mind and body.

Reducing stress

We are at epidemic levels of stress in our society. This is the result of many factors including, but not limited to, higher costs of living, longer working hours, cuts to support services and issues with family members and friends, amongst many, many other factors. Stress can negatively impact moods, our state of wellbeing, behaviour and health (Schneiderman, Ironson and Siegle 2005). Stress is not something we can get rid of completely; there will be points throughout our lives where we will have to deal with one or more stress factors.

What we do have control over, however, is our response to stress and what we perceive a stress to be. One way to reduce stress is to stimulate our parasympathetic nervous system (PNS). The PNS is essentially our destress button. When our PNS is triggered, our heart rate and breathing slow down, our intestinal and gland activity increases, our gastrointestinal tract relaxes and so does our mind. In contrast, when we encounter a stress factor, we stimulate our sympathetic nervous system (SNS), or our 'fight or flight' mode. When our SNS is triggered, our hypothalamus sends messages to release cortisol and adrenaline to increase our heart rate and blood pressure, and release sugars in the form of glucose to fuel our muscles and our mind, which can leave us feeling anxious or stressed. Our fight or flight mode, our SNS, can be triggered by a real or imagined danger, and it is there to keep us safe. For example, we could feel the fight or flight mode triggered if we see a tiger on the loose, or have a near-miss crossing the road. The increased heart rate, blood pressure and release of glucose would help us run away from the tiger or get across the road safely. But it can also be triggered when there is no real danger, just a perceived one. For example, you could be sitting in a coffee shop and all of a sudden you feel anxious, your heart rate increases, and you feel as though you need to leave immediately. There is no real threat, no tiger at the door, but your body is sending you signals that you are in imminent danger. This is because we can imagine threats – our mind creates them. This could be due to stress from rush hour traffic, our subconscious picking up on something it perceives could be dangerous, or it is reminded of a past danger or even the thought of a dangerous situation. The more time we spend in our fight or flight mode, the quicker and more easily we can get there. The more regularly we are stressed and are perceiving or imagining dangerous situations, the more time we spend in our fight or flight mode. This creates a vicious cycle and will have negative effects across all areas of our lives. However, the more time we spend in our relaxed state, with our PNS stimulated, the more resilient we are to life's stressors. The more time we spend in a relaxed state, the less likely we are to get stressed and trigger our SNS, our fight or flight response (Gard *et al.* 2014).

There are many ways to stimulate our PNS. Deep breathing, walking in nature, yoga, meditation and guided meditation are just a few. Any activity or thought process that calms down the body and mind stimulates the PNS, which makes us more resilient to the everyday and bigger stresses in life. By using guided meditation in a yoga class, you are offering your students a little pocket of peace; a calm, safe space to stimulate their PNS so they can enjoy the relaxing sensations on the mat, but also carry the benefits with them off the mat, out into their daily lives.

Creating a calm and productive workplace

A study found that just 15 minutes of guided meditation in the workplace could improve psychological and physiological symptoms related to stress. By introducing this practice the study also found that guided meditation enhanced job satisfaction and productivity (Melville *et al.* 2012). It shows that even short guided meditations have benefits that can permeate across all activities of the day, therefore making any jobs or tasks you need to do at work or home more satisfying and less stressful.

Increasing compassion

Self-compassion is an integral element in our sense of confidence and wellbeing, although it can be challenging to cultivate self-compassion when we are in a state of repetitive, negative thought cycles. A study has found that an effective way to break this destructive cycle is a guided meditation with the theme of self-compassion, and that just by listening to positive self-compassion meditations we can change our view of ourselves. A study involving a group of women with body dissatisfaction found that after three weeks of self-compassion guided meditation, they experienced significantly greater body appreciation, reduced body shame and improved self-worth. Wonderfully, all improvements were sustained when the group was reassessed three weeks later (Albertson, Neff and Dill-Shackleford 2014).

Compassion towards others can also be enhanced with guided meditation. Participants took part in a three-week study listening to compassion-themed guided meditation. The participants who listened to the guided meditation were shown to be more compassionate to a stranger in need of help than the group who had not taken part (Lim, Condon and DeSteno 2014).

By offering students themed guided meditations that focus on cultivating a certain trait, emotion or feeling, we can tailor the students' experiences to generate positive states that can improve their relationship with themselves and with the wider world.

Better sleep

Lack of sleep can affect a person's life in a profoundly negative way. Sometimes we struggle to get to sleep because of our 'monkey mind' worrying about things; or sometimes we don't get the chance to sleep as much as we need, as in the case of sleep-deprived parents and menopausal women. The amount of time that students are in a very deep state of relaxation as a result of guided meditation is four times as restful as that amount compared with sleep. So, if your students are in a guided meditation for half an hour, it has the same effect on their bodies and minds as two hours of deep sleep

(Saraswati 1976). This makes guided meditation a more effective and efficient form of rest for body and mind than conventional sleep. It helps us switch off from our monkey minds and find some respite, and recharges our energies, making it a nourishing practice for people who are sleep-deprived.

Guided meditation has been shown to benefit our physical body and our minds in a multitude of ways. By offering guided meditations in a class setting you are allowing your students to access these benefits on the mat and to continue to experience the multilayered holistic benefits off the mat too.

When to use guided meditation in a class

Guided meditations are generally used at either the beginning or end of a class. They can, of course, be used in the middle of a class, although this may disrupt the energetic flow of a yoga class. If you consider it in terms of when the best time is for your students to relax, the beginning and end of a class seem like the most natural places for rest, with the *asana* or *pranayama* work in between.

Beginning

When students arrive at the class it is beneficial for them to relax for a short period of time. This allows them a mental shift of focus, from the awareness being mostly based in the mind, their thinking state, their *manas* state, to drawing the awareness back into the body and the breath, their *being* state, to prepare them for the practice. Therefore, a short guided meditation is best for the beginning of a class, of around 5 minutes. If it is too long, the students may become too relaxed, and rousing them from a deep slumber may be met with some resistance.

Middle

If you choose to use a guided meditation in the middle of a class, the best time for this is usually after the supine warm-up, so more towards the beginning half than the end half of a class. This really depends on what type of class you are planning. Generally, yoga classes are planned as an arc, with a relaxing beginning building steadily up to a physical peak and then slowly coming back down to a relaxing end. In this case, the middle of a yoga class is generally where we work on the physical practice including *asana* and sun salutations. Therefore, it would be at odds with the pace of the class to put a relaxation guided meditation in the middle of a class. However, if you are planning a restorative or relaxing class, with very little *asana* practice, then the guided meditation could be seen as the peak of the class and would work well in the middle. The meditation can be done in a seated position (*sukhasana*) so the students will not become too relaxed or sleepy.

End

If your aim for a guided meditation is for the students to access the most relaxed state possible, then choosing to place the guided meditation at the end of the practice is best. The students will be able to fully relax and let go, knowing that the *asana* and *pranayama* practice is behind them. A study found that relaxation after a combination of yoga poses allowed the students to access deeper levels of relaxation than a guided meditation with no prior *asana* practice (Telles, Reddy and Nagendra 2000). Students can allow their awareness to be fully absorbed in the imagery of the guided meditation if it is at the end of a class, safe in the knowledge that nothing more is expected from them, and that they can completely let go and have a more immersive experience. This therefore makes the guided meditation more effective, embedding the theme or message deeper in the students' psyche.

Setting

There are many factors to consider when choosing the correct setting to hold a yoga class and guided meditation. The main aim is for the students to feel comfortable and to be in a safe environment. The points below outline the different elements to keep in mind.

Type of establishment

There are many different places you can hold a yoga class. A yoga studio is, of course, one of the most common. Gyms, community centres, school halls, church halls, village halls and home-based yoga studios are just a few other options. Any room that is large enough to hold a class and offers the additional amenities listed below will suffice.

Size and space

First, check if the space is the right size for you. You will have in your mind how many students you will be happy to teach. If the room is already used to teach yoga, ask the hirer how many mats they usually fit in the space. Ideally, it's good to offer each student at least 3–4 foot by 7–8 foot of space (around 1 metre by 2 metres). Also consider the size in terms of voice projection – could your voice be heard comfortably at the back of the room?

Check for coat hooks and shoe racks and if there are any places to store valuables, or whether the students need space for bags next to their mats for keeping valuables safe. The last thing you want is for students to worry about the safety of their personal possessions during a relaxation session. Check that there are enough coat hooks; in winter, if you have a class of 20 students, you need a lot of space to store all the coats, hats and scarves.

Facilities

To make your class as accessible as possible, ask the hirer if the room comes with car parking spaces and if so, how many. If not, check if there is a public car park nearby and if there is a charge so that you can pass this information on to your students. If there is no car parking, which is often the case in cities, check where and of what type the nearest public transport is.

It's always good to check the toilets yourself to see if you think they are acceptable and if there is a disabled option. Ask if there are changing rooms, which are not necessary but are a bonus, and whether the room has access to drinking water; if not, you can advise students to bring their own water bottles.

Health and safety

Ask the hirer about the fire exit, escape routes and the last time they checked that the fire alarms were working. Most spaces should carry out weekly fire alarm tests, so you should also ensure that a test alarm isn't due to go off in the middle of your session! Familiarise yourself with the escape routes and the meeting point outside, and share this information with your students.

Make sure you know where the first aid kit is and also where the nearest defibrillator is.

Look around the room and see if there is anything that could potentially fall on your students in a class. Community centres or similar settings often have stacks of chairs or white boards, amongst other objects, that could be a potential hazard.

Check that the space is adequately clean and there are no bad odours or signs of damp.

Props and equipment

If you hire a space or are employed by a yoga studio, you will undoubtedly have access to bolsters, blocks, blankets, cushions, eye pillows, straps and spare mats. Check with the hirer if you have permission to use the props if hiring from a studio. Access to props is a great bonus when teaching in a yoga studio as props can be expensive to buy as well as being tricky to carry around, as they are bulky. If you are teaching in a regular space that is not a yoga studio, see if there is a cupboard or storage space you could use to store your props, even if it's just a few mats, because undoubtedly, a few students may forget to bring mats or new students may not yet have a mat of their own.

Light

Check the natural and artificial light in the room. For guided meditation it is ideal to have a dimmer switch to create a soft light, so when it is time for the students to close their eyes, they will not be distracted by a bright overhead light. If the overhead lights only have an on or off switch and you are teaching in the day and there are windows, this may not be a problem as the natural light will be enough. However, if you are teaching when it is dark outside, you will need to consider other ways to bring a soft light into the space. Bringing a lamp could work, although carrying a lamp to every class along with your mat, etc., can be cumbersome. Another option is to offer your students eye pillows to place over their eyes if you need to keep the overhead light on.

If there are skylights, in the summertime you may need to offer students a place away from where the direct light lands on the floor. As I have found with skylights in the summer, students who lie in the sunny patch can often overheat, and when it's time for lying down and closing their eyes, it is uncomfortable for them to have the bright light in their eyes.

It is always a bonus to have some natural light and air in a room; check you can easily open and close the windows for ventilation in the summer. Basements always feel a little gloomy, but if this is your only option, they can be lifted with good lighting and a sunny teacher!

It is possible to create a soft light with candles, but if the space you are teaching in has a no naked flames policy, LED tea lights are a good alternative.

Heat

For students to comfortably relax in a guided meditation the room must be warm. If the students are cold, they will naturally feel uncomfortable and the focus will be on their discomfort and not the meditation. If you feel the room is a little chilly before you are about to begin your meditation, ask the students to put on socks, jumpers or to cover themselves with a blanket. You may also like to offer this option if you are using a guided meditation at the end of a yoga class, as the students would have become quite warm with the physical practice, but will cool down quickly when they lie still.

Check where the thermostat is and ask to be shown how to turn the heat up or down. Ask if the heating will be turned on and the room already warmed before you arrive in the colder months. Similarly check that the room has sufficient ventilation so it doesn't get too hot in the summer months. If the room relies on a fan, make sure it is not too noisy; and if it relies on the windows opening, check the windows can open and also that, by doing this, you are not inviting any sounds or air pollution into the room. Unwelcome smells, especially cooking or smoke smells, will negatively affect your students' experience, as will loud traffic or passing noises.

Time

Most rooms or studios for hire offer the room at an hourly rate, with 15 minutes prior to the start of the class to set up and 15 minutes after for your students to leave and for you to pack up. Double-check how much time you have before and after the class. See if there is a class booked in directly after yours and always endeavour to finish on time, as you never know your students' plans for the rest of the day.

See if you can visit the room at the time of day when your class will be held. This will allow you to check any noise or other disturbance that wasn't present when you visited the room the first time. I have known yoga teachers to book a class only to turn up on the day and find that a very loud martial arts class happens at the same time next door, or it's next to a busy bar that was shut in the daytime when they visited.

Price

Always be clear on the price and how and when the establishment wishes to be paid. This may be in cash weekly or by direct debit monthly or by bank transfer. Always get a receipt and invoice from the room hirer so you can claim it back on your tax return if you are self-employed. Similarly ask how much notice you would need to give them if you wanted to stop hiring the space. It is best to get this information in writing, via email, so you can refer back to it if necessary.

Sound

Check the acoustics of the room and the sound system if you are choosing to use music. Ask to be shown how to connect to the sound system and if the venue has a Music Licence. Be aware of noises outside the room to see if you think this may be a disturbance to the class. If the room is in a shared building, ask if any noise will be coming from the surrounding rooms at the time that you teach. The ideal space will have no sound disturbances, so the students will have no distraction in terms of sounds in the meditation, but if you are teaching in a city or town, this may be an impossible ask. If this is the case, a little background street noise is to be expected, and as your students will most probably live in the city or town, they are most likely used to these sounds and will not notice them or be particularly bothered by them.

To summarise, these are the basic factors to consider when looking for a setting in which to hold a class:

- Male, female (or mixed gender) and disabled toilets.
- Fire exits, escape routes and working fire alarms.
- Car parking or close to public transport links.
- First aid kit.
- Space for shoes, coats, scarves and bags.

- Safe space:
  - No mould.
  - Clear space, no objects that could fall on students, e.g. stacks of chairs.
  - No unpleasant odours.
  - Ventilation.
  - Adequate heating.
  - Adequate flooring.
  - Enough space for the maximum amount of students.
  - Clean.

Extra factors to consider:

- Access to drinking water.
- Changing rooms.
- Music system.
- Adjustable lighting.
- Access to props.
- Lack of sound pollution.
- Lack of air pollution.
- Natural light.

Positions for meditation
Student safety

Your main priority when teaching is to keep your students safe. With this in mind, always ask your students to fill out a questionnaire before their first class with you, with a section asking if they have any medical conditions or injuries, if they are on any medication, if they are pregnant, or if there is anything else you need to know about. Ask at the beginning of every class if your students have any new injuries or health concerns, and allow time to talk to them and offer any modifications necessary.

Sukhasana

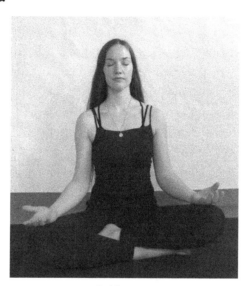

Sukhasana

Pronounced *suk-ah-sana*

Sukhasana is one of the main and easiest positions to meditate in from the possible options given in yoga. *Sukh* means 'easy', 'sweet' or 'pleasure' in Sanskrit, and 'sukhasana' is referred to as 'easy sitting pose' in English. However, unlike the name suggests, sitting in the pose for any length of time can feel far from easy. Therefore *sukhasana* is best used for short guided meditations and short *hasta mudra* meditations.

Benefits

- Allows a relaxed, yet alert, mind.

- Builds strength in the back.

- Opens the hips.

- Options for different hand positions.

Verbal cues for sukhasana

From a comfortable seated position:

- Slightly move the weight of the body a little to the left, to the right, to the front and to the back. From these slight movements find the point where you feel centred, where the top of the spine is directly above the base of the spine and you can feel a clear, straight line of energy.

- Place the hands on the knees with the palms facing up or down.

- Take a little lift through the crown of the head.

- Lift the heart and allow the shoulders to fall away from the ears.

- Relax the knees and let the inside of the thighs soften.

- Relax the belly.

- Settle into your seat.

- Feel a connection with the root of your being.

- Become aware of the opposing forces as you sit: the force of gravity gently grounding you to the earth, and the slight lift of the crown connecting you to your higher self.

Modifications and props

If the knees are higher than the sit bones, place a block or two under the sit bones until the knees and sit bones are the same level.

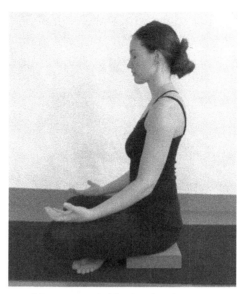

Sukhasana modification with block to level the knees with the hips

If there are any problems with the knees, place a bolster lengthways down the mat and kneel on the bolster. This will take any weight-bearing pressure off the knees.

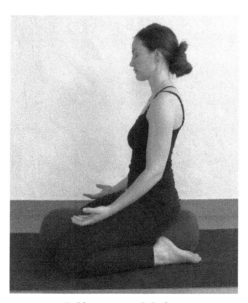

Sukhasana with bolster

For older students or those with reduced mobility or flexibility, offer a chair if *sukhasana* is not an option. Ask them to sit with a straight back, feet hip-width apart and flat on the floor.

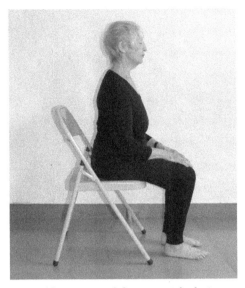

Sukhasana modification with chair,
for students who cannot access a seated Sukhasana

Shavasana

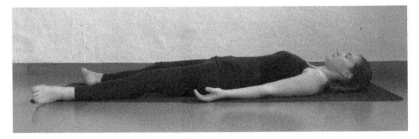

Shavasana

Pronounced *sha-VAH-suh-nuh*

Shavasana (from *sava*, corpse), known in English as 'corpse pose', is the main *asana* in yoga for full body and mind relaxation. It is the perfect position for students to do the short or long guided meditations in, although the intention is not to fall asleep; rather, the intention is to reach a state of waking relaxation. Offer the students the option of raising an arm if they feel as though they are drifting off.

Once in position it is beneficial to keep the body completely still, to allow the muscles and the mind to reach the deepest level of relaxation available.

Benefits

- Releases muscular and skeletal tension.
- Develops body awareness.
- Slows down breathing and the heart rate.
- Restores and revitalises body and mind.

Verbal cues for shavasana

From lying down:

- Take your ankles to the edges of the mat and allow the feet to fall away from each other.
- Deeply relax the knees and the thighs; let them roll out.
- Soften into the hips; let them gently open.
- Take the arms down by the sides of the body, with the palms facing up.
- Shuffle the shoulder blades back and down.
- Slightly tuck the chin into the chest and lengthen through the back of the neck.
- Take a deep breath into the belly; breathe into the tops and sides of the lungs.
- Have a sense of releasing and letting go on the exhale breath.

Modifications and props

The neck should be in line with the spine, so offer students a thin block or folded-up blanket or pillow to place under their neck.

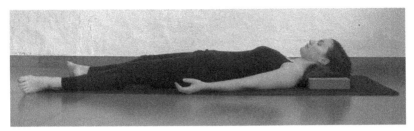

Shavasana with block under the head to bring the head and spine in line

If the student has issues with the lower back, offer temple pose as an alternative, as this takes a little pressure off the lower back. Temple pose: Lie on your back with your knees bent and the arms down by the side of the body with the palms facing up. Walk the feet to the hip bones or as close as feels comfortable for you. Then step the feet slightly wider than hip distance apart. Slightly tuck the chin in to the chest and relax the shoulders back and down.

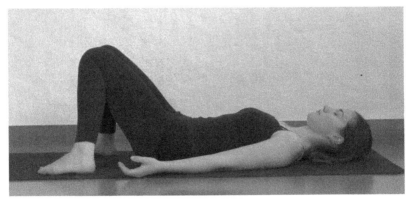

Temple pose modification for lower back pain

Alternatively, offer a bolster under the knees or a chair to rest the lower legs on.

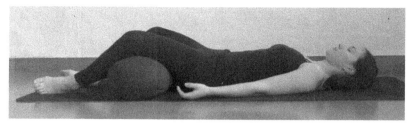

Shavasana modification bolster for lower back pain

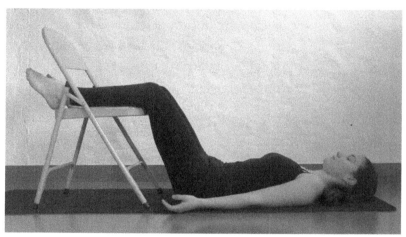

Shavasana modification with chair for lower back pain

Adaptations for pregnant students

There are two options if teaching students who are pregnant:

- Side-lying *shavasana*: Ask your student to lie on their side with a blanket under their hip for extra padding, if needed. Place a block between the knees or rest the top knee on a bolster. The knee and hip need to be the same level, so add a blanket or any extra padding on top of the bolster if needed. Rest the head on the inside of the bottom arm or block, and rest the top arm on another bolster.

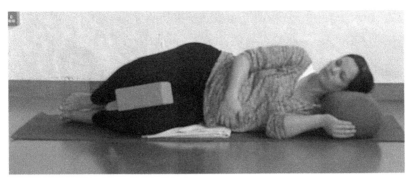

Shavasana modification with props for pregnant students

- *Sukhasana*: Place blocks under the sit bone so the knees are the same level as the sit bones. Hands can be placed in any position, although, when pregnant, it makes a nurturing connection to place one hand on the heart and one hand on the belly.

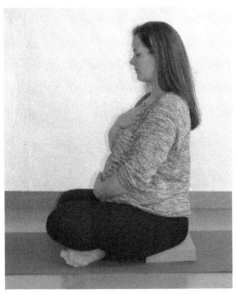

Shavasana modification with block for pregnant students

Voice

True voice

It may seem obvious, but speaking in your own voice is best for guided meditation. Although this can feel like an unusual point to make, sometimes, when we teach yoga, our voice changes. Our accent may shift slightly, we may take the same tone as a hypnotist or any other such change in our voice. This may be due to lack of confidence in our own voice or feeling that we need to step into character before we teach. The result may be a voice that doesn't sound natural or true. Students can pick up on this shift of voice; it is easier for them to relax fully in a safe environment with an honest, true voice. From a *chakra* perspective, the voice is linked to the *vishuddha chakra* and it is most open and true when we are naturally ourselves. Remember, your magnificence shines brightest when you relax into your natural self.

Tone

Our natural voice has many different tones. The tone we use in a guided meditation will be different from the tone we use when we are teaching *asana* or *pranayama*, which will be clearer, a little louder, and possibly more assertive. For guided meditation use the same tone as you would if you were reading a child a bedtime story – a calm, peaceful tone, layered with a loving kindness.

Volume

The volume needs to be loud enough so the voice is clearly projected across the entire room, yet still keeping the tone soft. If you choose to use music, check it is low enough so your voice can be heard comfortably above the music. It is surprising, in a silent class, how low the music can be, yet it is still heard by the students. If you are playing music as the students arrive, with the hustle and bustle of unpacking mats and settling in, when the class has settled and the students are silent, the music can be turned down. If there are any students with hearing problems, make sure they are at the front of the class.

Silence and time

Embrace the silences and pepper them throughout the guided meditation. As a teacher it can feel uncomfortable leaving silences, but these are the moments when the students can fully absorb what you're saying. They can paint vivid pictures in their minds to amplify the experience. These are the moments where your words are interpreted and realised in the student's mind's eye; allow them the space to delve into their own pools of expression.

The length of the silences can extend as the meditation continues. At the beginning you may leave a gap of one round of breath (e.g. four seconds in and out) between each line in the script, and then maybe two rounds of breath; you may even work slowly up to leaving a full minute of silence if you have reached the peak of the meditation, to allow the students to become fully absorbed in the imagery you have handed them, but always consider the time. The longer meditations in this book can be anywhere from 5 to 15 minutes long, depending on the speed at which they are read and the silence allowed in the spaces. It is always ideal to finish a class on time. You never know what plans or commitments your students have after the class, and if they sense that the class has run over, it will make them feel agitated. Therefore, always keep one eye on the clock, and make sure you have time and adjust the length of silences accordingly.

Music

Music is not necessary for guided meditation and is one of those things that is totally up to the teacher's discretion whether to include it or not. There are arguments for and against its use. Some teachers prefer not to use it for a number of reasons. It is seen as honouring the more traditional lineages of yoga to not use music. Music to accompany a yoga class is never mentioned in the *Hathayogapradipika* or Patanjali's *Yoga Sutras*. Sound is mentioned in Chapter 4 of the *Hathayogapradipika*, but it relates to *nada*, which focuses the internal sounds of the body as a way of gaining *samadhi* (pure consciousness). It is thought of in some traditional lineages of yoga that music itself is a distraction. Iyengar considers music in a class as distracting 'fluff'. But guided meditation, discarding yoga *nidra*, is not part of the traditional lineage.

On the other hand, music can be seen as an aid and not a distraction in a yoga class as it can instantly set the mood for the practice. It has the power to enrich the atmosphere and make the guided meditation a more immersive experience. It is especially useful for students who are new to yoga or new to guided meditation to anchor their awareness into the room and to stop mental distractions.

Whether you choose to use music or not is entirely up to you. You must do what resonates most soundly with yourself. Try not to consider what your students would prefer as you cannot please everyone. If you stay true to your style of teaching, then you will attract the students who resonate with you, and all that is wonderful and unique about you.

Music Licence

If you choose to play music in your lesson, in the UK, you or the venue will need a Music Licence. The venue you teach in should have their own Licence, and if they do, you will not need one; but it is always best to check if they have the Music Licence, which consists of the PPL (Phonographic Performance Limited) Licence and PRS (Performing Right Society) for Music Licence. Gyms, health clubs, yoga studios, church halls and community centres should all hold an up-to-date Music Licence. Previously venues and teachers had to purchase a PPL Licence and PRS Licence separately, but now the organisations have come together to form the PPL PRS Music Licence, and you can find information and buy a personal Licence from them if you need one from their website.[1]

Volume

One of the main factors to consider is the volume of the music. The volume level is integral for the music to not become a distraction and for its main purpose to be background music. Set the level after the class is silent and the students are in the position they will stay in for the guided meditation; this may involve turning the volume down just before you are to begin your guided meditation, as it may have been set a little higher for the previous part of the class. You do not want your voice competing with the music.

Type of music

There are a few factors to consider when choosing a piece of music for a guided meditation.

Lyrics

It's best to choose music with no lyrics so the students' awareness has only one 'voice' to listen to. Two voices, yours and the singer's, with two different subject matters, may become confusing and a distraction for the students. The only time that music with lyrics seems to work is if the lyrics are not in students' native language. For example, a piece of music with some gentle chanting of mantras in Sanskrit may not distract – the chant becomes part of the music as the student cannot understand the words.

Pace

Background music tends to work best if it is slow-paced. Your students will be in a relaxed position, the breath and heart rate will have slowed down, so to mirror this, the music must be slow and at a gentle pace.

---

1   See https://pplprs.co.uk

Genre

Considering the above point about pace, this cuts out many genres of music – drum and bass or a lively jazz piece would contradict the mood. The obvious choice is a type of New Age music or some sort of instrumental music like singing bowls. Classical music or a piece of piano or guitar music with a gentle melody also works well. The genre must also be one that is generally well received. Too niche, and there is more chance that some students may not like it. Remember that the music in a guided meditation is there for background mood setting and is not the main event.

CHAPTER 2

Short Guided Meditations for the Beginning of a Class

Using a short guided meditation at the beginning of your yoga class allows your students to mentally arrive for the practice. It allows them the space for a mental shift from the awareness of being in the mind, from their thinking and doing state, to adjusting to the pace and tone of a yoga class. Just a short 5-minute guided meditation can begin to relieve some muscular and mental tension and set up the right frame of mind so they can fully access the benefits of the yoga class.

These six meditation scripts are all designed to quickly but gently transfer your students from the state they arrive in to a relaxed and receptive one. The meditations focus on tried and tested methods of achieving this, by reconnecting with the breath, the sensations in the body, relieving muscular tension and promoting positive emotional states.

Short guided meditations are best used at the beginning of a class as the aim is to relax the students just enough to relieve any held tensions or stress they have carried from their day to the class, but not enough to send them into a deep relaxation so they feel sleepy, which would not be ideal for the upcoming physical practice of the class.

Take your time when reading the scripts. There is no rush, and don't be scared to leave spaces of silence to let the students fully experience their meditation journey. As a yoga teacher, sometimes we feel we must talk a lot to guide our students, which, of course, in most instances, is the case, especially with *asana* practice. But it is in the spaces of silence that the students can fully realise and have the space to interpret and embody the themes of the meditations.

Sun rising (5 minutes)

This meditation uses the imagery of a sun rising in the heart to reignite the student's wonder and excitement for this one precious life we have been gifted. Sometimes we become numb to the monotony and routine of life, and this meditation acts like a little spark to awaken our curiosity and enthusiasm. It is an uplifting and energising meditation, perfect for the beginning of a class.

Take your time reading it. Allow the spaces of silence to extend slightly as the meditation continues. The pace of the meditation is meant to mirror a sunrise, a slow, gentle beginning to relax the student. Then the momentum and inspiration build like an arc, before slowly coming back down. By the end, the student should feel relaxed but with a rejuvenated sense of wonder about themselves and the world again.

*Note: Each bullet point represents a round of breath. Use this time to read the next line in your mind so when you read it out loud it flows naturally. The ** symbol represents a longer silence.*

The students can be in either *shavasana* or *sukhasana*, depending on your preference for these meditations. You can use the verbal cues found on p.24 and p.27 as a script to guide the students into these positions before beginning the short guided meditation script:

- Drop the focus to the heart space.

- Allow a breath to be felt here.

- Bring a hand to rest on the heart.

- Adjust the touch so it is light, a nourishing gesture.

- Begin to tune in to the energy being released from the palm of the hand.

- Notice the exchange of heat from the palm of the hand, warming the heart.

- Allow the heart to respond to the warmth of this connection.

- Let it soften and expand.

- Give it permission to open, open to care, open to love.

- Now imagine a tiny drop of golden light falling from the centre of the palm into the centre of the heart.

- From this tiny speck of glistening light a sunrise is born.

- Feel the sun rising in your heart.

- An optimistic sunrise bathed in the excitement of a new day, new beginnings, brightening and widening your horizons.

- The warmth of unconditional love and self-confidence is woven on the beams of light that spread in all directions.

- Casting light, excitement and inspiration to the dawn of this new day.

Leave a silence of a few rounds of breath here

- The rays of pure energy move up into your mind, switching on a child-like sense of wonder in the world again.

- The golden beams move down into your belly, igniting a courage and strength to carve out your own path.

- The sunrise grows brighter, filling your arms and legs in preparation for the upcoming adventure that is your one wild and precious life.

Leave a silence of a few rounds of breath here

- The light brings a glow to your face.

- It moves into and illuminates all the cracks and corners of your being.

- The rays of light begin to draw back to the heart now.

- But tiny flecks of golden stars are left glistening around the body.

- The sparks to light the flame of your next adventure.

To close the class (1 minute)

Use this short script if you wish at the end of the class to link back with the theme of the meditation:

- Come back to the sunrise in your heart.

- Visualise it there now.

- Feel the sense of wonder and excitement its energy brings.

- Notice the flecks of shimmering light, gleaming all around you.

Observing the breath (5 minutes)

Pranayama is generally defined as breath control, although in reality it is much more than this. *Pranayama* uses the breath to influence the flow of *prana* (our life force). The first stage of *pranayama*, before we begin any breath manipulation, is to become aware of the breath. Sometimes we spend an entire day, week or month without even noticing the breath or the way we breathe. This is a simple guided meditation designed to allow the students just to become aware of the breath and the way we breathe. It begins with full deep breaths to relax the students, and is an obvious vehicle to feel the sensations of the breath. It then moves to the subtler qualities of the breath and allows the breath to move from the chest, where it is sometimes held. The meditation then turns into more of a mindful practice, trying to keep the focus on the soft breath and not letting the mind wander. It's a lovely simple meditation to start the class, and will release tension and bring about awareness of the breath that will benefit the students' experience of the class. As stated in Patanjali's *Yoga Sutra*, 'The experience of asana requires an appropriate effort, the relaxation of all unnecessary tensions and a constant awareness of the flow of breath' (2.47, Taimni 1972).

Note: Each bullet point represents a round of breath. Use this time to read the next line in your mind so when you read it out loud it flows naturally. The ** symbol represents a longer silence.

The students can be in either *shavasana* or *sukhasana*, depending on your preference for these meditations. You can use the verbal cues found on p.24 and p.27 as a script to guide the students into these positions before beginning the short guided meditation script:

- Take a full breath into your belly.

- Exhale slowly to release the breath.

- Now this time, really become aware of the sensations in your body as you breathe.

- On the inhale, feel the rise of the belly, the slight stretch of the skin.

- On the exhale, feel the deflation of the lungs and the belly.

- Take two more full rounds of breath like this, anchoring the awareness to the sensations in the body as you breathe.

- And when you have finished your two rounds, release the breath around the body into a natural rhythm.

- Allow the breath to move where it needs to go.

- Soften the diaphragm so the breath has free reign to move where it wants to, down to the legs or up to the shoulders.

- Allow the breath to breathe itself.

- No effort is required.

- Just watch how the exhale ends and, with no effort at all, the next inhale begins.

- For the next few rounds of breath just watch for this magic moment, when the exhale naturally extinguishes and the new inhale is created.

Leave a silence of a few rounds of breath

- If the mind wanders, that is fine. That is what it does. Just gently guide it back to where we want it to be, observing the breath.

- Check that your face is relaxed, your jaw is soft and your eyebrows released. Sometimes when we are concentrating, the body and face tense.

- Release any held tension on your next exhale.

- Then see if you can release another layer of tension on the next exhale.

- Imagine every exhale feels like a light veil is being lifted away from the body, releasing another layer of tension.

- Deeper and deeper you relax.

- Heavier and heavier the body rests on your mat.

Leave a silence of a few rounds of breath

- Take one last full deep inhalation into your belly, and exhale slowly to release.

- Come back to your body and where it rests in the room.

During the class

Remind your students to come back to the breath throughout the practice, especially in the more challenging poses where it is easier to hold the breath. Remind them to keep it flowing at a natural, steady speed. If you have introduced your students to *ujjayi* breath, remind them to keep the gravelly, wave-like sound flowing.

Setting an intention (5 minutes)

Setting an intention for a yoga class is to bring your attention to a quality you would like to cultivate more of. These intentions can sometimes be qualities that the student can extend off the mat and use in their daily life, thus promoting the concept that the benefits of yoga are not just confined to the mat, and that it is an holistic practice that permeates all areas of our life.

Choosing an intention can be quite daunting and it is normal for the student to struggle to find the clearest, deepest reason for them being at the class. So, in this meditation, we create a link with our subconscious mind via the third eye to call on our intuition to guide us in choosing the intention. The meditation has been left void of any suggestions about what the intention may be, so as not to influence the student's choice in any way. This is to promote the space for the most honest and personal intention to arise.

*Note: Each bullet point represents a round of breath. Use this time to read the next line in your mind so when you read it out loud it flows naturally. The ** symbol represents a longer silence.*

The students can be in either *shavasana* or *sukhasana*, depending on your preference for these meditations. You can use the verbal cues found on p.24 and p.27 as a script to guide the students into these positions before beginning the short guided meditation script:

- Observe the point between the eyebrows.

- Let it soften and expand.

- This is the point of your third eye.

- Your centre of intuition.

- An energetic gateway that transcends our conscious mind and communicates with all the realms of our being. Connecting ourselves to our higher self. Our wisest, truest self.

- Notice the quality of the energy at this point between the eyebrows.

- Can you feel a tingling here?

- Does it have a colour?

- Now ask your intuition the question, 'What is the deepest intention for coming to the practice today?'

- What was the primal driving force that drew you to your mat today?

- Allow your intuition to answer.

Leave a silence of a few rounds of breath here

- It may come quickly; it may take a while.

- Just wait and see what surfaces.

- Whatever rises up out of the depths of your intuition, just observe it.

- Let it float there.

- Hold it in the space it needs.

- Then ask yourself, 'How can I incorporate this into my practice today?'

- It may be something physical to work on. Or something on a subtler energetic level.

- Now draw this intention, like a jewel from your third eye, and place it in your heart space and give the heart permission to hold your intention throughout the practice today.

During the class

Come back to the intention a few times throughout the class if you wish. A good time for this would be when the students have their hands in *anjali mudra* (prayer position, see p.62) with the backs of the thumbs resting on the heart. You could remind them:

- Take a moment to reconnect to the intention you set at the beginning of the practice and realign with your practice to honour the intention.

Or:

- Check in with your intention. Your jewel nested in your heart space. And ask, how can it guide you through the rest of your practice today?

To close the class (1 minute)

Use this very short script if you wish, at the end of your class, to close the practice and link back to the theme of the meditation:

- Come back to that intention you set at the beginning of the class.

- Your precious jewel, nestled in your heart space.

- See if you can hold it there and carry it with you off your mat into your day. A glistening spark of intention from the depths of your intuition, guiding you through your day.

Letting go (5 minutes)

Sometimes students arrive with baggage. This can be stresses from work, responsibilities or baggage they have put on themselves with negative thought patterns. This 'letting go' meditation allows students to unburden themselves from this baggage, and by doing so, begin the process of releasing tension. This meditation uses guided visualisation, which is a powerful tool in transformation, to assist with the students letting go so they can fully arrive, mentally and physically, for the class.

*Note: Each bullet point represents a round of breath. Use this time to read the next line in your mind so when you read it out loud it flows naturally. The ** symbol represents a longer silence.*

The students can be in either *shavasana* or *sukhasana*, depending on your preference for these meditations. You can use the verbal cues found on p.24 and p.27 as a script to guide the students into these positions before beginning the short guided meditation script:

- Become aware of yourself, resting here, in this space.

- Allow yourself to fully arrive on your mat.

- Sometimes our physical bodies are on our mats, but the mind is elsewhere.

- Maybe it's wandering into the future, planning for the rest of the day. Or reliving a moment that has passed.

- But remember, this is your space, right here, in this present moment.

- Your sacred space in your waking day, where you are free from all responsibilities and pressure.

- Imagine nothing exists outside of this room.

- In here you hold no external titles or pressures that come with these. For the length of this class, nobody needs anything from you. There are no emails to answer, people to look after or jobs to be done.

- Here you can rest in the freedom of just being you.

- Imagine placing anything that happens outside of this room in a box.

- Place your chores for the rest of your day, your stresses, your grievances, your shopping list.

- Put your desires, your goals, your motivation to change yourself in any way. Put the steam that powers your engines towards the targets you've set for yourself in your box.

- With intention, place all pressures, slight or big, positive or negative, in your box.

- Put the thoughts that wake you up in the middle of the night and the manic energy that drives you down the road to your greatest, fullest self in your box.

- And when you have laid them all to rest in your box, set the lid down, wrap it up with a ribbon and leave it just outside the studio door.

- Now rest in the space that is left behind.

Leave a silence of a few rounds of breath here

- You are perfect just as you are in this present moment.

- Accepting yourself fully in this precious moment.

- Allow the body to adjust to this.

- Maybe the shoulders can sink a little deeper.

- The legs may be able to roll out a little more.

- The belly can relax and expand a little further.

- How does this precious gift of space feel when it is held only for you and your needs?

- Take a long, soft inhale into this space.

- With a sigh, slowly exhale.

- Take one more round of breath like this.

To close the class (1 minute)

Use this short script, if you wish to close the class, as an extension and to link in with the meditation:

- Don't forget to pick up your boxes that you left outside the room at the beginning of the class.

- Take a moment to cherry-pick the items you want to take with you. Choose anything that will lift and bring light into your life or the lives of the ones you love.

- Leave behind anything that seems too heavy to carry now.

Cleansing breath (5 minutes)

A cleansing breath is a great way to allow the students to release any held physical or emotional tension. We use the guided imagery here of a wave of light, moving through the body with the breath, as a way to clear out anything that the student is ready to let go of. The result is a lighter feeling, physically and mentally, that will improve the physical quality of the upcoming class and their mental quality off the mat.

*Note: Each bullet point represents a round of breath. Use this time to read the next line in your mind so when you read it out loud it flows naturally. The ** symbol represents a longer silence.*

The students can be in either *shavasana* or *sukhasana*, depending on your preference for these meditations. You can use the verbal cues found on p.24 and p.27 as a script to guide the students into these positions before beginning the short guided meditation script:

- Soften the awareness to the soles of the feet.

- Feel the bottom of the toes, the curve of the heel and the lift of the arch.

- Notice the line that separates the sole of the foot from the air.

- Feel the temperature of the air against the sole.

- Now allow this boundary line to slightly blur.

- As if a connection has been made.

- Take the focus to the crown of the head now.

- Again, noticing the line that separates the crown of the head and the atmosphere above.

- Letting this line slightly blur as if a connection has been made.

- We are going to take a few rounds of a cleansing breath.

- On the inhale, imagine inhaling through the crown of the head. Drawing a cleansing breath down through the body from the top of the head to the soles of the feet.

- On the exhale, release through the soles of the feet. Letting go of anything that no longer serves you.

- Keep the breath natural.

- Like a soft wave flooding the body from head to foot.

- Feel the inhale drawing light through your entire being.

- Feel the wave of light washing out anything heavy, any debris you've collected.

- Feel the release through the soles of the feet.

- With every breath you feel lighter. Brighter.

Leave a silence of a few rounds of breath here

- Take one more full inhale and releasing exhale.

- Allow the crown of the head and the soles of the feet to gently close.

- Become aware of the line that separates them from the atmosphere.

- Hold the light within you.

To close the class (1 minute)

You can use this short script if you wish to close the class:

- Just come back to that sensation of light we cultivated within you earlier, with the cleansing breath.

- Just tap back into that now.

- A brightness, shining through your being to all corners of your body.

- As you leave the class today you leave bathed in the light of your own magnificence.

Body scan (5 minutes)

A body scan is a great meditation to do at the beginning of a yoga class, as it allows the students to reconnect with their physical bodies, which will aid and deepen the experience of the upcoming *asana* practice. Body scans have been popularised by mindfulness as they are a very simple but effective meditation to shift from a busy thinking mind on autopilot to a calm focused mind, using the physical sensations of our body as an anchor for the awareness to keep coming back to. It's this repetitive anchor of gently drawing the focus back to the physical sensations of the body every time the mind naturally wanders off that builds up the meditation muscles in the mind.

Body scans can also help with stress levels and our emotions. Sometimes it's only at the end of the day or when we explode with anger or stress that we really realise how much pressure we have been under. Without reconnecting back to our physical self, we can be unaware that we are near to our limit. The body scan allows us to access early warning signs of tiredness, stress or tension in a relaxed state, and by doing so, release the muscular and emotional build-up of tension, therefore allowing us to carry on the day more relaxed but also more in tune with our wellbeing, and more able to reduce the build-up of further tension.

*Note: Each bullet point represents a round of breath. Use this time to read the next line in your mind so when you read it out loud it flows naturally. The ** symbol represents a longer silence.*

The students can be in either *shavasana* or *sukhasana*, depending on your preference for these meditations. You can use the verbal cues found on p.24 and p.27 as a script to guide the students into these positions before beginning the short guided meditation script:

- We begin by taking a body scan of your internal landscape and how that looks and feels today, in this present moment.

- As we scan, make no judgements on what you find, and we are not going to change anything. We are just honestly checking in with how we feel today.

- Observing and just noticing the sensations in the body.

- Begin by noticing the feet, dropping the awareness to the opposite end of the body. We spend so much of our days in our minds, let's really feel the feet right now. What do you find here?

- Drawing the awareness to the interior of the feet. How do they feel? Name the sensations. Can you feel any tingling? Slight movements of energy? Or maybe there is nothing, just a numb sensation?

- Now draw the internal gaze to the legs. Notice the full volume of the legs. How do your legs feel?

- If they can relax a little deeper, give them permission to rest a little heavier, let them roll out.

- Feel the torso now. With a sense of curiosity, like you are discovering a new place, scan from the pelvis up to the shoulders, and just see what you find here, in this moment.

Leave a silence of around five rounds of breath here

- If the mind has wandered, that's fine, that's what it does. Just gently guide it back to where we want the focus to be right now, in the torso.

- Adjust the focus to your arms now. Feel your awareness filling the space from your shoulders to your fingertips.

- Notice the quality of the energy you hold in the palms of your hands today.

- Move the focus to your head now. Inhabit the full space in the head, from the crown of the head, to the base of the skull.

Reach the awareness to the sides of the head, noticing the space between the ears.

- Widen your lens to your entire body as a whole now.

- And when you are ready, come back to the breath.

- Take a full inhalation into your belly, and exhale slowly to release.

CHAPTER 3

Hasta Mudras

Hasta mudra is translated as 'hand gestures', *hasta* meaning 'hand' and *mudra* meaning 'gesture', 'seal' or 'attitude'. The *Kularnava Tantra* traces the word *mudra* back to its separate meaning of *mud*, 'delight' or 'pleasure', and *dra* from *dravay*, which means 'to draw forth'.

Hasta mudras work with *prana* (life force/energy) and can redirect this life force back into the body via the hands. In yoga it is believed that the *nadis* (invisible channels that carry our *prana* around our bodies, similar to meridian lines) constantly radiate *prana* and this *prana* is usually lost from the body. By using a *hasta mudra* it creates a kind of circuit that can loop the *prana* (the life force) back into the body. Different *hasta mudras* enhance and promote different qualities, for example, *chin mudra* connects us to our higher selves. *Hasta mudras* are a great vehicle to get your students to access the subtler energetic levels of their practice and become aware of their *prana* and the rejuvenating effects when it is redirected. *Hasta mudras* also serve as a physical way to monitor our focus when meditating, as when we lose the focus and the mind wanders, the hand releases from the *mudra*, making *hasta mudras* an aid to extending concentration in meditation.

Position

For *hasta mudras* it is best to sit in *sukhasana*. Refer to p.24 for verbal cues and modifications. As *sukhasana* can be challenging to sit in for a long time, unless you are an experienced yogi, these *hasta mudra* scripts are around 5–10 minutes long.

Chin mudra (5–10 minutes)

Pronounced *ch-in*

Chin is derived from the word *chit* or *chitta*, which means 'consciousness', and links us to our higher consciousness. It is one of the most recognised *hasta mudras* and can be held in two ways. The first is with the tip of the index finger connected to the tip of the thumb creating a circle, which is the position we will use in this meditation. Holding the *hasta mudra* this way allows the student to become clearly aware of the circuit that is created when we hold *chin mudra*, looping the *prana* back into our bodies, up to the mind, and connecting us with our higher state of consciousness.

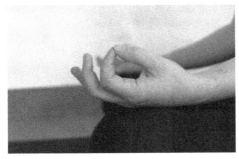

Chin mudra with tip of index and thumb connected.
Links us with our higher consciousness

The second way to hold the *mudra* is by connecting the tip of the index finger to the root of the thumb. The three relaxed fingers, the middle, ring and little finger, represent the three *gunas*, the three qualities of nature: *tamas*, stability; *rajas*, activity and creativity; and *sattwa*, harmony. For our consciousness to transfer from ignorance to knowledge we must surpass these states. The index finger represents our individual consciousness, *jitvatma*. The thumb represents higher consciousness. So in this *hasta mudra* the individual (index finger) is bowing down to the higher consciousness (thumb). The fingers are touching, symbolising that although the individual is acknowledging the power of the higher consciousness, there is a link and a unity of both through yoga.

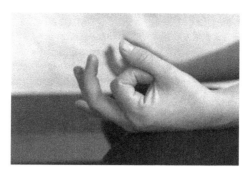

Chin mudra with tip of index and root of thumb connected.
Links us to our higher consciousness

This guided meditation works with this idea that we are linked to our higher selves. It is designed to promote confidence in our knowledge of ourselves and to create a connection with our higher self so we seek guidance from our innate knowledge when needed.

Settle your students into *sukhasana* using your own verbal cues or those found in the *sukhasana* script on p.24.

*Note: Each bullet point represents a round of breath. Use this time to read the next line in your mind so when you read it out loud it flows naturally. The ** symbol represents a longer silence.*

- Rest your hands on your knees with the palms facing up.

- Close your eyes.

- Drop your awareness to the tip of the index finger and the tip of the thumb.

- Just notice the sensations there.

- Keeping the awareness here, connect the tip of the index finger and the tip of the thumb.

- What do you notice at this connection point?

- You may notice a slight or apparent transfer of energy.

- You may notice nothing at all, just a numb sensation, and that is fine. This is your own unique experience. We are just observing what is there.

- *Chin mudra* creates a circuit to loop *prana*, our life force, which is usually lost through the hands, back into the body. This particular *mudra* loops the *prana* back up the inside of the arms to the brain, and connects us with our higher consciousness. This may be felt very subtly or quite clearly.

- It lifts dull energy and gives us clarity of mind, like the transformation of a muddy pool to crystal clear waters.

- Tap into the connection between yourself and your higher consciousness now.

- Your highest, wisest, kindest self.

- Picture yourself sitting here now, in your mind's eye. Sitting exactly as you are in the clothes you are wearing, holding your hands in *chin mudra*.

- Now picture your highest self, sitting opposite you, like a mirror image.

- An image of your highest, wisest, kindest self.

- And you feel as though you are sitting opposite an elder, someone whose opinions and guidance you know is true and you trust.

Leave a silence of a few rounds of breath here

- Sometimes we look to others for advice: loved ones, strangers or even celebrities.

- We listen to his solution or hers, and they are sometimes very helpful.

- But there is another option, another source of knowledge, where we sometimes forget to look.

- And its unique solution is only one you can see.

- Sometimes we spend so much time and energy looking outwards, but if we took a moment to look internally, we would find the answer and the guidance we seek is already here.

Leave a silence of a few rounds of breath here

- We hold an innate, ancient knowledge about ourselves. We know deep down what is best for us.

Leave a silence of a few rounds of breath here

- Come back to that image of your highest self now and know that it is you.

- Next time you are struggling with something, take this *mudra*, sit with yourself and look to your highest, wisest, kindest self for guidance. The connection has been made and will always be there. Come back to yourself to find the solution you seek.

- Trust in yourself.

- Believe in your instincts.

- Everything you need is already here.

- Come back now to the tip of the index finger and the tip of the thumb.

- Just notice the quality of that connection, that exchange of heat and energy now.

- And when you are ready, take a full breath into your belly and open your eyes.

Anjali mudra (5–10 minutes)

Pronounced *ahn-juh-lee*

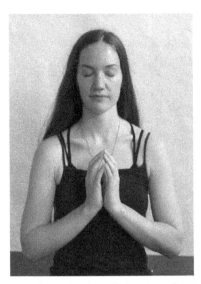

Anjali mudra 'to offer' or 'to salute'

Anjali mudra is one of the most common *hasta mudras* used in a yoga lesson; so common it has its own emoji. *Anjali* translates from Sanskrit as 'to offer' or 'to salute'. In this meditation we will be offering the heart a blessing.

There are two ways to hold this *mudra*. The first is with the palms of the hands flat against each other. The second is with the fingers slightly bent, so there is a gap between the palms of the hands. For this meditation we will use the second option, which allows the students to access the physical sensations of *prana* relating to this *mudra*.

*Note: Each bullet point represents a round of breath. Use this time to read the next line in your mind so when you read it out loud it flows naturally. The ** symbol represents a longer silence.*

- Connect the palms of the hands. Connect the tips of the fingers and the outside edge of the thumbs, keeping a slight bend in the fingers. There should be a slight gap between the fingers. Rest the backs of the thumbs against the sternum, in the heart centre and close the eyes.

- Take a few deep breaths.

Leave a silence of a few rounds of breath here

- Allow the breath to settle and let it move around the body.

- Draw the awareness to the tips of the fingers.

- Feel the exchange of heat, of energy between the tips of the fingers.

- Notice the space between the palms of the hands.

- Acknowledge any sensations here.

- You may feel a slight buzz of energy, you may be able to feel a presence, it may have a certain colour.

- There is magic in this place.

- Held in this space between the palms.

Leave a silence of a few rounds of breath here

- Visualise this *prana*, this energy, as a shining light, filling the space between the hands.

- You may be able to feel its physical presence filling the space. Maybe you can feel its warmth?

- Now watch as the light begins to beam in between the gaps of the fingers, spreading out in all directions.

- Some of this light shines directly into the heart.

- Just allow the light to enter the heart space right now.

- Feel it expand and open the chest.

- Connecting with your heart space and its needs.

- Visualise the heart as a vast sky.

- Abundant.

- It holds a rainbow of emotions.

- Ask your heart what needs attention right now.

- What needs care or love.

- Offer your heart a blessing.

- Offer it a blessing based on what it needs at this moment.

Leave a silence of 30 seconds here

- Draw the awareness back into the tips of the fingers.

- Notice the breath.

- Breathe slowly and deeply into the heart.

- Gently open the eyes.

During the class

Try using *anjali mudra* as we used it in the meditation, with the fingers slightly bent and a gap between the palms of the hands, throughout the class. It can be used in any pose and is especially effective in sun salutations as it brings a softer, more attentive, quality to the salutations.

Kali mudra (5–10 minutes)

Pronounced *k-uh-lee*

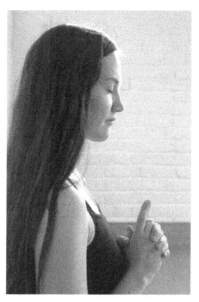

Kali mudra to empower and build inner strength

Named after the fearsome goddess Durga, *kali mudra* is a powerful *mudra* that promotes courage, builds strength and empowers us to stand in our own truth. The fingers are interlaced with the left thumb on top of the right to represent a feminine quality, as the left side of the body is thought to be more dominated by female energy. The two index fingers are then extended with the fingertips touching, to represent the sword of Durga who slays illusions.

This is a meditation for self-empowerment and self-confidence, a way to reconnect with our inner strength that is always there, though sometimes forgotten or lost.

*Note: Each bullet point represents a round of breath. Use this time to read the next line in your mind so when you read it out loud it flows naturally. The ** symbol represents a longer silence.*

- Bring the palms together at the chest.

- Cross the left thumb over the right and continue until all fingers are crossed.

- Extend the index fingers, so the fingertips touch. This represents the sword of Durga, who slays illusions.

- We will use this *mudra* to lift the veil of negative illusions we have about ourselves and build our inner strength.

- Tap into these stories we tell ourselves, the veils of negativity that cover up our true strength and inner greatness.

- Illusions of negative thoughts.

- Illusions of self-doubt.

- Illusions of fear.

- As these veils lift, we peel back the layers and uncover who we are at our core.

- Our true self resides here.

- Our raw, primal force of nature and strength reside here.

- This strength may feel quite apparent; it may feel easy to connect with.

- Or your inner strength may feel quite small right now, like a little seed.

- No matter the size, it is there.

- As our heart lies in our chest, our inner strength is at our core.

Leave a silence of a few rounds of breath here

- Use the inhalation to build your inner strength.

- Like stoking the flames of a fire.

- Or encouraging an ember to glow.

Leave a silence of a few rounds of breath here

- Let the warm, fiery energy move from your core and begin to spread around your body.

- Drawing courage to the heart.

- Wisdom to the mind.

- And strength to stand in your truth and shine in your unique magnificence.

During the class

Link the meditation into the class by using *kali mudra* in poses. The hand position can be used in Warrior 1, a low lunge or standing position.

Padma mudra (5–10 minutes long)

Pronounced *pud-ma*

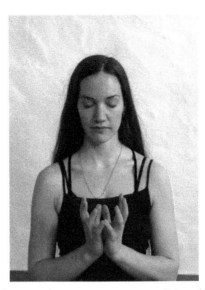

Padma mudra to promote unconditional love

Padma translates as 'lotus', and this *mudra* represents the lotus flower and the blossoming of unconditional love for ourselves and for others. Just like the lotus flower sits on top of muddy waters, unconditional love blooms above the muddied feelings of fear and loneliness. This meditation promotes the blossoming of unconditional love for ourselves and for others as a blessing we can give and receive.

Settle the students into *sukhasana* (see p.24) or any other comfortable seated position.

*Note: Each bullet point represents a round of breath. Use this time to read the next line in your mind so when you read it out loud it flows naturally. The ** symbol represents a longer silence.*

- Bring the hands into prayer position, resting on the heart.

- Take a moment to connect with your heart space. Feel the backs of the thumbs rest on the heart centre, forging an energetic connection, a gentle opening.

- *Padma mudra* represents the blossoming of unconditional love for ourselves and for others.

- Come into the *mudra* by keeping the connection with the palms of the hands, the tips of the thumbs and the tips of the little fingers, and gently unfurl, separating the three middle fingers.

- Notice the blossoming sensation in the hand and the mirroring sensation in the heart, opening to love.

- Allow space in the heart for this unconditional love to bloom.

- We are not covering anything up, just allowing the space that it needs.

- Just as the lotus flower floats on top of the muddied water of fear and loneliness. We are not denying those feelings are there. Allow them space to be there. Just noticing that love can transcend and blossom above these feelings.

- Picture the face of someone you love in front of you. Look into their eyes.

- Feel their presence in front of you.

- Now offer them a blessing of unconditional love, by whispering their name in their ear, saying 'I love you' and embracing them with a hug.

- The more you connect with the physical feeling of the hug, speak their name, pass on the words, the more powerful the blessing will be.

- Now see them looking into your eyes, whispering your name, hear them say, in their tone of voice, 'I love you'. Feel their blessing of unconditional love pass to you as they hug you.

- Notice the connection of love and how the heart naturally opens to this.

- Feel the sensations of the warm embrace.

- Fully receive their blessing of love.

- As you fully give your blessing of love.

- An open field of connection.

Leave a space of around 30 seconds silence here

- When you are ready, gently draw the fingers back together and hold the image of the lotus flower in the heart.

Hridaya mudra (5–10 minutes)

Pronounced *hrih-day*

Hridaya translates as 'heart', so we can look at the *mudra* as a heart gesture. This *mudra* works with established energy channels (*nadis*) to create a direct link to the heart. This *mudra* has a cleansing and revitalising quality that can lift feelings of a heavy heart. It is a great *mudra* to use when going through an emotionally challenging time to unburden the heart and lift the spirits.

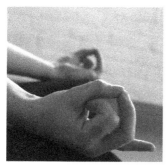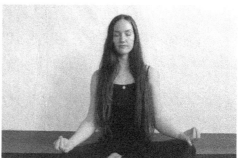

Hridaya mudra links to the heart and revitalises the body

Settle the students into *sukhasana* (see p.24) or any other comfortable seated position.

*Note: Each bullet point represents a round of breath. Use this time to read the next line in your mind so when you read it out loud it flows naturally. The ** symbol represents a longer silence.*

- Connect the tip of the index finger to the root of the thumb. Join the tips of the thumb, middle and ring finger. Straighten up the little finger and have the palms facing up.

- Close the eyes and just connect to the circuit that's been created.

- This *mudra* diverts *prana*, our life force, to the heart *chakra* (*anahata chakra*), improving vitality and unburdening the heart of any heaviness.

- The middle and ring fingers connect directly to the heart via the *nadis*, the pathways that carry the *prana* around the body.

- The thumb acts as an energiser and creates the circuit to divert the flow of *prana* from the hands to the *nadis* in the middle and ring finger, so they can carry this energy direct to the heart.

- Just tap into this circuit now.

- Notice the flow of energy running down the middle and index finger, travelling up the arm and flowing into the heart.

- It carries a light energy to lift the heart.

- As we hold this *mudra* we allow the heart, just for a few moments, to unburden itself, to gift it some breathing space. Sometimes we carry so much in our hearts. Let us unload for a few moments and see how this feels.

- Picture a heart-shaped box in your mind.

- Lift the lid gently and just peer inside.

- What do you find there?

- Is it busy and full, or is it quite empty?

- You can picture anything in your heart as an object.

- Choose one thing now you would like to take out of your box. Something that has been weighing you down. Something that has been a burden on your heart. Maybe a conflict with a loved one or a hurtful memory.

- Intuitively see what form this takes and carefully lift it out of the box and set it far away.

- How does that feel? Does your box feel a little lighter? Does it look a little less cluttered?

- Now continue to remove objects from your box. Name them. Note the form of the object and with a sense of ceremonial attention, remove it from your box.

- And notice how much lighter it feels. Every time an item is taken out, notice how much lighter your box becomes.

Leave a space of silence here

- When you have taken your last object out of your box, just peer back inside. Notice what you have kept in there. What do these objects look like? What do they represent?

- Your loved ones.

- Your passions.

- Your precious memories from happy times.

- Carefully place the lid back on your box.

- Take a deep breath into your belly, exhale slowly to release, and when you are ready, open your eyes.

Yoni mudra (5–10 minutes)

Pronounced *yon-ee*

Yoni translates as 'womb' or 'source', and the diamond shape created by the index finger and thumb represent the womb. However, this *mudra* is not about creating feminine energy. It actually promotes a balancing of energies by interlocking the fingers, and uses a 'seed' energy from connecting the thumb and index finger to power this process. This guided meditation uses imagery of a control panel in a tree to balance the emotions and energies of the body.

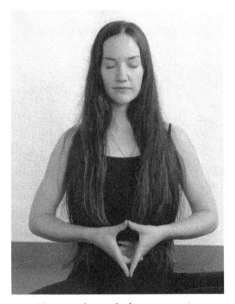

Yoni mudra to balance energies

Settle the students into *sukhasana* (see p.24) or any other comfortable seated position.

*Note: Each bullet point represents a round of breath. Use this time to read the next line in your mind so when you read it out loud it flows naturally. The ** symbol represents a longer silence.*

- Bring the hands to prayer position at the belly. Interlace the middle, ring and little finger. Keep the tips of the index fingers connected and the tips of the thumbs connected. Point the index fingers down and point the thumbs up.

- Take a full inhale and on the exhale, close the eyes.

- Settle into the sensations of the *mudra.*

- The interlaced fingers create a cross connection of energies from left to right and vice versa.

- This crossing of energies flowing back and forth balances the energies of the body and also brings balance to the right and left hemispheres of the brain.

- The connection of the tip of the index finger and the tip of the thumb powers this flow of *prana*, this flow of energy.

- Just notice the contact point between the tips of the index fingers and the tips of the thumbs now.

- You may notice a circuit-like flow of energy.

- *Yoni* refers to the womb or the source.

- By holding this *mudra* we reconnect with our primal source energy and use this to bring balance to our bodies and minds.

- This balance can be represented by a tree.

- Picture in your mind's eye a tree.

- Allow your intuition to present you with a tree.

- What does your tree look like? Notice the leaves. The branches.

- The trunk of your tree. And as you look at the trunk, you notice a door.

- Walk towards the door in the trunk of your tree.

- Feel the sensation of the bark on your hands as you gently open the door.

- Inside the tree you see a control panel.

- There are lots of dials and at the top of the control panel your name is written.

- As you look a little closer at the dials you notice each dial has a word written above it.

- All the dials have different words written and they all relate to emotions.

- There is happy, sad. Angry, calm. Content, restless. Stressed, relaxed.

- Each dial is set somewhere between high and low. There is a balanced point at the centre of the dial.

- Just take a moment now to gaze across your control panel and see where your dials are set.

- Notice the ones that are high. Notice the ones that are low.

- You can take some time now to readjust your dials to a setting that you choose.

- Kinaesthetically feel your hand turn a dial up or down to fully engage with the balancing process.

- If stress is too high, turn it down.

- If creativity is too low, turn it up.

- So just take some time to adjust your dials.

- When we sit with this *mudra* we invoke our primal seed energy to power this balancing process.

Leave a gap of silence of a few rounds of breath

- Just make those last few adjustments now.

- And when you are happy, leave your control panel and close the door of the tree.

- Allow yourself just to sit and be for a few rounds of breath, just letting everything reset. Realign.

- Take a full inhale of breath into the belly and as you exhale, gently open the eyes.

- Release the hands from the *mudra* and rest your hands in prayer position at the heart.

CHAPTER 4

Longer Guided Meditations

This chapter covers longer guided meditations to be used at the end of a class. A longer guided meditation can benefit the body and mind in a few ways. The first is by releasing tension. A lot of us move through our day holding on to tension that we are completely unaware of. Sometimes our shoulders are hunched up towards our ears, or our belly is tense and held. Just notice in yourself now. How does your belly feel? If it's a little tense, take a few deep breaths and then see how it feels. Tension can be held anywhere in the body: in the neck, the thighs, the chest, etc. A longer guided meditation has the time to release these layers of tension to allow the body and mind to truly relax in ways that other relaxing activities may not. If you were to ask someone what they do to relax, they may say that they watch TV or scroll through social media or read a book. Although these activities may give pleasure and other benefits, they are not truly relaxing in the sense of releasing tension. Take watching a TV drama, for example. When we watch TV, although we are sitting down, our body and mind are not relaxing. Our mind is being stimulated by the images and the storyline and, in turn, our body tenses and goes through an emotional journey with the characters. Have you noticed before when a character is in a car chase, for example, and you are willing for them to be free from their chaser, the stomach tenses, cortisol is released and your breathing is shallow? Rather than relaxing, the body and mind actually create more tension.

Guided meditation is one of the best ways to bring the body, breath and mind back into balance. It's a way of releasing the built-up tension that we have created over the day or the week and not carrying it over into the next day. This has a multitude of benefits: it lowers stress, helps us relax and sleep better; it allows a busy mind to slow down; it releases physical tension; it regulates our breath. And when the body does all these things, life itself seems better overall. If we are less stressed, we are less likely to get stressed. When we tune back into the physical sensations of the body, we promote better physical health because we can listen to the messages the body is sending us. Life seems to flow more easily because we are relaxed and going with the flow, not carrying our tension with us.

A longer guided meditation gives your students space to unburden themselves from the stresses, worries and responsibilities of their everyday lives. It is a practice in self-care, a way for them to access a deep level of relaxation and all the benefits that come with that. Each of the meditations in this chapter has a separate theme and promotes cultivating a different positive emotional or physical state.

Sun meditation, a healing meditation (10 minutes)

This meditation uses the imagery of a healing orb of light that floats around the body providing relief and a healing energy. Even though each bullet point represents a round of breath, you can use your intuition, and leave a longer silence to let your words sink in. This meditation begins with a short relaxation to release tension by allowing the students to focus on different sensations. The more relaxed they are, the more effective the imagery of the meditation will be.

*Note: Each bullet point represents a round of breath. Use this time to read the next line in your mind so when you read it out loud it flows naturally. The ** symbol represents a longer silence.*

Begin by settling your students into a comfortable position. If you choose *shavasana*, use the *shavasana* script on p.27 if you wish:

- Take a full breath into your belly, and a long exhalation to release.

- Keep the breath as soft as you can this time; inhale softly and fully into the belly. And with a sense of release, exhale.

- One more time. Inhale softly, fully into the belly. With a sense of sighing and letting go, release on the exhale.

- Release the breath around the body. Allow it to flow and move naturally. Let the breath breathe itself. No effort is required.

- Just notice the face. Allow the face to fully relax. Notice the point between the eyebrows and let it soften. Smooth the brow. Relax the jaw.

- Notice the connection of the lips and the sensations in the mouth. Release the tongue from the roof of the mouth and relax down to the root of the tongue.

- With every exhale, the body rests a little heavier on your mat.

- You relax, let go a little more.

- As if you are held by your mat, held in the space.

- Tune into the energy in the palms of the hands.

- Begin to draw in the energy from the sun into the palms of the hands: draw it in through the windows, the door, from the light in the room around you.

- Gather this up until you have a glowing orb of light in each palm.

- This is a pure light. A healing energy. One of our primal energies.

- Lift the hands and interlock the fingers. Rest the hands on the heart. Feel the two orbs merge into one as they gently sink into the body.

- Feel this pure energy, this healing orb of light, glisten softly in the heart space.

- This orb has the power to heal anything it comes into contact with.

- Let this orb float around the body, let it go wherever it needs to go. It will intuitively move to a certain part of the body where it will heal in whatever way is needed. It may release tension, it may give unconditional love, it may relieve a heavy weight.

- You do not have to do anything, the orb's intuition will connect with the body's intelligence and they will work together to heal.

- When the healing is complete it will move on to another area.

- Follow this orb. Let it be your guide around the body to other areas that need healing, where it will shine its light, heal and nourish the area before moving on.

- Feel the presence of pure healing light.

Leave a silence here of around a minute

- It may move to parts of the body that surprise you.

- It may go somewhere familiar.

- Embrace and accept its journey and allow it to heal.

- Give your body permission to heal.

Leave around a minute's silence here

- Now bathe the entire body in this healing light.

Leave a 30-second silence here

- The light begins to shrink back into the heart space.

- It slowly lifts out of the body, back into the palms of the hands.

- Place your hands down by the sides of the body, holding your orbs.

- Release the sunshine energy back into the room.

- Become aware of the light within.

- Slowly come back into the room and where your body rests in the space.

- Gently shake your head from side to side.

- Bring a little movement into the fingers and toes.

- Stretch out in any way that feels comfortable for you right now.

Watching thoughts, a calming meditation for the mind (10 minutes)

This meditation sets up this concept of 'observing' in the relaxation. The observing in the relaxation is focused on the sensations in the body as a way of focusing the mind and setting up a non-judgemental and unattached attention. The landscape of the body is then swapped with the imagined landscape of the mind, and the student can practise a simple meditation of being separate from their thoughts. This is a calming meditation to disconnect, for a few moments, from the constant stream of thoughts, and to just become the observer.

*Note: Each bullet point represents a round of breath. Use this time to read the next line in your mind so when you read it out loud it flows naturally. The ** symbol represents a longer silence.*

Begin by settling your students into a comfortable position. If you choose *shavasana,* use the *shavasana* script on p.27 if you wish:

- Take a full breath into your belly. Lengthen the breath on the exhalation.

- Soften and lengthen the next inhale. Breathe deeply, softly, into the bottom of the belly; now draw the breath into the upper lungs. With a sense of letting go, exhale slowly.

- One more round of breath like this, being fully present with the sensations of the breath.

- Release the breath around the body into a natural rhythm.

- Become aware of your body, resting in this space.

- Let yourself fully arrive.

- Allow the eyes to soften and the brow to smooth.

- Drop the awareness to the solar plexus, that point just below the ribs but just above the belly button. Drop the focus deeply at this point. Let it open and expand. Give it the space it needs.

- Adjust the internal gaze to take in the body as a whole now.

- Become aware of the *prana,* your life force moving around the body. Just tap into those sensations now. Notice any tingling. Any slight movements of energy. Drop into those sensations of your body on an energetic level.

- Scan down from your head to your feet. Scanning and tuning into the energy frequencies present in your body today.

- Making space for whatever you find.

- Not to cover up or ignore anything that's there. Just watching and observing. With a sense of curiosity about what you find.

- Your wonderful landscape. Your unique ecosystem.

Leave a silence of at least 30 seconds here

- Imagine you are sitting at the top of a hill.

- It's a beautiful day and you can see a vast landscape in front of you.

- You look at that point where the land meets the sky. The blur of the horizon. So far away. The blurred line of the horizon feels like it is of this world and then also like it is not. Like looking at a dream or a memory.

- Notice the great expanse of blue sky. Dotted with a few clouds.

- Your thoughts are the clouds.

- Separate from you, yet created by you.

- Watch them with curiosity.

- Name the thought that you notice on your first cloud.

- It's like you don't even need to think it; it is just there.

- What is that thought?

- Watch it like an observer.

- Detached from the emotional connection to it. Detached from it completely. So far away from it. Free to really see it for what it is.

- Watch it with no judgement. Just a child-like sense of curiosity. Like an investigator.

Leave a silence of at least 30 seconds here

- Move the gaze to another cloud.

- What is that thought?

- Name it. And again, with a detached sense of curiosity, just observe it.

- Does this thought relate to the past? Or to the future? Is it a thought you've had before?

- Is it a true thought? Or is it just your perception of reality?

Leave a silence of about 30 seconds here

- Move the gaze to one more cloud. Investigate it. Where does this thought come from? Is it a new thought or a well-known one?

Leave a silence of about 30 seconds here

- Come back to the sensations of sitting on top of the hill. Gazing out to that vast blue sky and the clouds moving across the vast expanse. How does your sky look? Are there just one or two clouds or lots of clouds?

- No matter the amount. Right now, they are separate from you. Something happening far away.

- Feel the grass underneath you. Rest your hands beside you and fully connect with the experience of gently pushing your hands into the grass.

- Feeling grounded, connected to the earth.

- Imagine bending your knees and gently pressing your bare feet into the soft, warm grass.

Leave a silence of a few rounds of breath here

- Come back to your body now.

- Feel the parts of the body that are in contact with your mat.

- Feel the parts that slightly lift away from the mat.

- The waves of the body. Rising and falling, on and off the mat.

- Some parts connected. Some parts lifted.

- Notice the curve of the back.

- Grounded at either end of the spine and the gentle rise and fall in between.

- Just feel the sensation of this arc.

- Becoming aware of where the body rests in the room and the space around you.

- Take a full breath into the belly.

- Exhale slowly to release.

- Gently shake your head from side to side.

- Bring a little movement into your fingers and into your toes.

- Allow the body to stretch out or move in any way that would feel good right now.

- And when you are ready, open your eyes.

Springtime meditation, blossoming into your true self (10 minutes)

This is a lovely, optimistic, guided meditation that takes the students into springtime and harnesses the energy of new growth that spring brings. After a relaxation where the focus is placed on the soles of the feet, the students are transported to a garden in spring to connect with the nourishing and invigorating vibrations of spring sent up from Mother Nature. Allow the space of silence between each bullet point to become a little longer as the meditation progresses.

*Note: Each bullet point represents a round of breath. Use this time to read the next line in your mind so when you read it out loud it flows naturally. The ** symbol represents a longer silence.*

Begin by settling your students into a comfortable position. If you choose *shavasana*, use the *shavasana* script on p.27 if you wish.

- Relax into the space. Resting onto your mat.

- Take a full breath into your belly. Exhale slowly to release.

- Take another full inhale into your belly. Now breathe into the tops and sides of your lungs. And with a sigh, release on the exhale.

- One more breath like this. Breathe into your belly. Now draw the breath into the upper lungs, expand the breath sideways. And with a sigh, release on the exhale.

- Let the breath flow around the body in a natural rhythm.

- Relax the diaphragm to liberate the breath from the chest and give it permission to move freely.

- A gentle wave of breath, lapping over your body.

- Take the awareness to the soles of the feet.

- Notice how the sole of your right foot feels.

- Feel the bottom of your big toe. What do you sense there? Does it tingle? Does it vibrate a little? Or is there nothing? Does it feel numb? Just watch the sensations.

- Notice the bottom of the other four toes on your right foot. Do they all feel the same? Or different?

- Shift the focus now to the sole of the left foot.

- How does the bottom of your toes feel on this foot? Is it exactly the same as your right foot, or different somehow? Can you name the sensations you find there?

- Notice the lift of the arch of the foot. Watch the sensations of the arc of the arch. The sweeping lift and fall. Notice it on the right. And on the left. Does the arch of the foot feel the same as the toes or different?

- Widen the lens to the body as a whole now.

- Feel the touch of the air on your skin.

- Remember now the touch of the air in springtime.

- Cast your mind back to a springtime memory and how the perfumed scented air softly swept across your body.

- You are there now, in a garden. The flowers of spring carpet the floor.

- Just take a moment to enjoy their beauty.

- Under some trees you see a cosy bed on the garden floor, surrounded by these beautiful flowers.

- As you climb into the bed you notice how comfortable and soft it is.

- You rest your head on the pillow and look up through the gaps in the leaves to speckles of sunlight and patches of the great blue sky beyond.

- You look around at the beautiful shades of the bountiful springtime flowers.

- Under the ground the energy of spring is stirring.

- A nourishing energy of new growth vibrates gently up from the depths of Mother Earth, calling to the bulbs to grow. To blossom.

- As you rest here, in your cosy bed on the garden floor, you begin to tune in to nourishing vibrations, the springtime energy sent up from Mother Earth.

- Align yourself with the vibrations of spring. Welcome them into your body. Let them pass through. Feel your body begin to wake up. Like little buds slowly opening.

Leave a silence of around a minute here

- An awakening energy. A fresh start.

- Let the waves of vibration power the new growth to unfurl.

- Feel the tingle of all the atoms invigorating the body.

- Hear the call from Mother Earth to you. To grow. To blossom into your true nature.

Leave a silence of around a minute here

- Slowly come back to yourself and where you lie in the space in the room.

- Gently shake your head from side to side.

- Bring a little movement into your fingers and your toes.

- Allow the body to stretch out and release in any way that would feel good.

- Take a full breath in and out.

- And when you are ready, open your eyes.

The open door, a meditation to welcome feelings and balance emotions (10 minutes)

This guided meditation uses a mindfulness technique to help balance emotions. It is the idea that if we welcome in all our emotions, the positive as well as the negative, we bring about balance. Sometimes we have the tendency to push negative emotions away if we don't want to feel them, but this just makes them stronger. This meditation uses the imagery of an open door to recognise and welcome the complex arc of emotions we encounter on a daily basis, and takes away some of the strength of the negative emotions. Ultimately, by letting them all in, we find balance.

*Note: Each bullet point represents a round of breath. Use this time to read the next line in your mind so when you read it out loud it flows naturally. The ** symbol represents a longer silence.*

Begin by settling your students into a comfortable position. If you choose *shavasana*, use the *shavasana* script on p.27 if you wish.

- Inhale deeply, filling the front of your body with a new breath. Exhale with a sense of letting go.

- On the next breath, inhale fully into the belly, the lower and upper lungs. Exhale with a sense of letting go.

- One last full breath, expanding the breath sideways. Enjoy the sense of release on the exhale.

- Then let the breath flow back into a natural, resting rhythm.

- See if you can let go a little more.

- Allow the face to relax. Let the legs soften and let the thighs roll out a little more. Feel the point in the centre of the throat open.

- Let those areas of habitual tension soften.

- Notice any areas of tightness, and just see if you can let them go, just a little more.

- Feel the shoulders float.

- Just floating. Nothing is holding them. Sense the space around them. Everything letting go.

- What happens to the shoulders when you let them float?

Leave a silence of around 30 seconds

- Imagine you are standing inside your own front door.

- Picture the door clearly in your mind's eye.

- You open the door and you see yourself standing there.

- It is a very happy version of yourself. You give your happy self a big hug and let them in.

- Then you see a very sad version of yourself come to the door. You give your sad self a warm embrace and invite them in as well.

- Next you see a very excited version of yourself come to the door. You give your excited self an enthusiastic hug and invite them in to your home.

- Looking up, you see a depressed version of yourself come to the door. With compassion you embrace and welcome this version in.

- Take some time now to welcome in all versions of yourself.

- Your entire rainbow of emotions.

- Name each one. See each emotion personified and arrive one by one at your door. The more you fully connect with the experience, each individual experience of welcoming in each emotion, the more you physically feel yourself embrace and welcome them in, the more powerful this becomes.

- Some may be easy to welcome. Some you may not want to welcome in at all. But if we ignore them, if we push them back, they will just keep coming back, fighting harder for our attention. If we recognise them, see them, greet them with open arms and welcome them in, then they pass, like a wave crashing on the shore. Strong at the time, but gone in a moment.

• Take your time now to name each one and just be curious, with no judgement, about who comes to your door today.

Leave a silence of a minute here

• When you have greeted the last few, you look around inside your house and see all the versions of yourself and you see balance.

• Your fiery self is teaching your shy self confidence. Your compassionate self is consoling your hurt self. Your calm self is soothing your angry self.

• When we recognise and welcome this vast rainbow of emotions, we find balance.

• There are no positive or negative emotions.

• They are all there to help us.

• Anxiety keeps us safe. It's a primal warning signal for danger. Next time you feel a wave of anxiety, just welcome it. Say, 'Hello there old friend', check to see if there is any obvious danger and if not, thank it for coming up, but tell it you are safe and then carry on with whatever you were doing. Welcome it in and it will pass. Try and push it away and it will keep knocking on the door.

• Life is an ocean and if we ride the waves, we will find the smoothest path.

• There will be highs and lows on the journey.

• Ride the highs and know that the lows will pass.

• If you ever need a *mantra* for the low moments, say this to yourself, 'This too shall pass'.

- Just think of the arc of emotions we pass through every day.

- They are all part of the great rainbow of life.

- The light, the dark. The yin, the yang. The sun and the moon.

- Open the door and you will find balance.

Leave a silence of around 30 seconds here

- Bring everything back into balance now by sending an inhalation down the central channel of your being, and exhale slowly to release.

- Gently shake your head from side to side.

- Bring a little movement into your fingers and your toes.

- Stretch out in any way that would feel good for you now.

- And when you are ready, open your eyes.

Waking up in five years' time, a meditation to reset your compass in the right direction (10 minutes)

This meditation allows the students space to imagine where they will be in five years' time. The positive imagery and content of this projection of their future self allows them to reset their internal compass to their chosen destination.

*Note: Each bullet point represents a round of breath. Use this time to read the next line in your mind so when you read it out loud it flows naturally. The ** symbol represents a longer silence.*

Begin by settling your students into a comfortable position. If you choose *shavasana*, use the *shavasana* script on p.27 if you wish:

- Take a full breath into the belly. Feel the breath received in the base of the belly. Slowly release the exhale.

- Keep the breath soft this time. Softly breathe into the base of the belly; now draw the rest of the inhalation into the upper lungs. With a sense of letting go, slowly exhale.

- One more breath like this. Softly, fully, breathing into the belly, now expanding the breath into the upper lungs. And on the exhale, being one with the sensations of letting go and release.

- Allow the breath to flow freely around the body now, in a natural rhythm.

- Relax the diaphragm and soften the belly to let the waves of breath wash fully over the body.

- See if you can let the full weight of the body rest a little heavier on your mat.

- See if the thighs can roll out a little more.

- Can the thumbs or the hands soften further?

- Check there is no tension being held in the forehead. Smooth the brow.

- Do any little adjustments you need to now, to release any held tensions.

- Notice the parts of your body that are in contact with the mat.

- Feel the backs of the heels rest on the mat.

- Notice the hips and shoulders.

- Become aware of the back of the head resting.

- Now notice the parts of the body that lift away and the space between your body and the mat.

- That space where the spine lifts and falls back onto the mat.

- The space where the back of the neck is not touching.

- And the space where the ankles lift off the mat.

- Just scanning and noticing the parts that are in contact with the mat and the parts that lift off.

- Notice the different sensations at these parts.

Leave a silence of a few rounds of breath here

- Take the awareness to the space where the spine lifts and falls from the mat. Just becoming aware, not of the spine itself, but of the space underneath. Can you feel the slight contact of the atmosphere nestling against the arch of the spine that lifts off the mat?

- See if you can make that atmosphere a little denser now, so you can feel it a little more. Like a fluffy cloud has come into that space and you can feel the cloud filling the area and slightly supporting the arch of your back. The touch is soft and supportive, as if you are being held by the cloud.

- Now imagine all the pockets of space where the body lifts off the mat, a cloud is now filling these spaces, offering a soft little lift, and the points of your body that are in contact with the mat feel a little lighter.

- The cloud begins to wrap around the sides of your body now and you feel its gentle support lift the outer edges of your body.

- Now it begins to move under the parts of your body that are in contact with the mat, so you begin to lift off just an inch or two.

- First one ankle lifts and then the other.

- The cloud moves under the arms and shoulders and they rise up a little too.

- The head feels weightless and free as it begins to be supported. Until the cloud has slowly moved under your entire body and you float.

- Your whole body just floating in space.

- Imagine now your whole body floating in space.

- You are surrounded by stars.

- Infinite space.

- Nothing is below you.

- Nothing is above you.

- Floating, safely, in the infinite universe.

- Surrounded by velvety blackness and glistening golden stars.

- Moving through time in space now.

- As you rest, floating in the stillness of the universe, the earth spins below you.

- It spins until it is five years in the future.

- Now your fluffy cloud moves back underneath you and delivers you back down to earth and into your bed. It is morning time.

- As you wake up, five years from now, what do you see? What does your bedroom look like?

- You can be anywhere in the world you want.

- Your bedroom can look however you want it to look.

- What do your bed sheets look like?

- What is the view from your window?

- Just take a moment to take in your room.

Leave a silence of a few rounds of breath here

- As you get out of bed and walk around the room, take it all in.

- And now it is time to get dressed.

- What clothes are in your wardrobe?

- It could be anything you want.

- Standing in front of the mirror now and looking at yourself, how do you look? What clothes are you wearing? What does your hair look like?

- Try not to overthink, just watch the images that pop up in the mind, like watching a film.

- How do you look? What emotions do you see in your face? Are you happy? Relaxed?

- How do you feel? Energised? Healthy? Balanced?

- Move downstairs to your kitchen now.

- And just taking a moment, take in your kitchen.

- Look all around. What does it look like?

- Sitting down at your table, look down at your list of things to do today.

- What is on that list?

- It could be anything at all. What activities would bring you most joy?

- Are you meeting up with anyone today? If so, who and what will you be doing?

Leave a silence of a few rounds of breath here

- It is time for breakfast.

- You can invite anyone in the world to your table. Who joins you? Or do you choose a quiet breakfast by yourself?

- What are you eating? It could be anything at all. Eggs from the chickens in your garden. A smoothie or porridge made by a loved one.

- Fully experience being at your table now. Sitting in your dream home, in your perfect kitchen, with your loved ones at your table. Feeling inspired and excited about the day ahead. Everything feels at peace. Everything is balanced.

Leave a silence of a few rounds of breath here

- Imagine closing your eyes at the table and now you are back, floating weightlessly in space above the earth as it begins to spin backwards, coming back to the present time.

- Hold on to that image of you at your table in five years' time and set your internal compass to that destination.

- Trust in the forces of the universe to guide you to this destination. It is not the final destination, just a pinpoint on the map of the journey in life.

- Feel the sensations of the cloud begin to gather beneath you.

- As it slowly and gently lowers you back down onto the mat.

- Again, become aware of the points of the body that are in contact with your mat.

- Feel the connection between the earth and your body, grounding you back into the space in this room.

- Take a full breath into the belly, and exhale slowly to release.

- And when you are ready, open your eyes.

If you choose to end the class by chanting 'OM', you can use this very short script to link the closing of the class with the meditation:

- Finish the practice by chanting 'OM'. Send this 'OM' through the passage of time to yourself sitting at your breakfast table in five years' time to create an energetic link from now to then. Exhale naturally now. Inhale deeply. 'OM'.

Chakra crystal meditation, to balance the chakras (10–15 minutes)

This meditation has more spaces of silence than other long guided meditations as the process relies on the students connecting with their inner sensations, which requires these breaks. This is a lovely meditation and results in feelings of balance and improved wellbeing by using the imagery of crystals and *chakras*.

*Note: Each bullet point represents a round of breath. Use this time to read the next line in your mind so when you read it out loud it flows naturally. The ** symbol represents a longer silence.*

Begin by settling your students into a comfortable position. If you choose *shavasana*, use the *shavasana* script on p.27 if you wish:

- Take a deep breath into your belly. Exhale slowly to release.

- In your own time, take three more rounds of slow deep breaths on the inhale and sigh on the exhale if there is anything that needs to be released.

Leave a silence of around three slow rounds of breath here

- Allow the breath to move around the body in a natural rhythm.

- See if you can relax and let go a little more.

- See if your thighs can roll out a bit more.

Leave a silence of two rounds of breath here

- See if the hips can softly open.

Leave a silence of two rounds of breath here

- Let a warm, relaxing sensation spread across the lower abdomen.

Leave a silence of two rounds of breath here

- Allow this warm, relaxing sensation to move up the belly to the lower lungs. Letting go, releasing tension.

Leave a silence of two rounds of breath here

- Allow the breath to be felt at the heart.

- Feel a sense of peace spread across the heart space.

Leave a silence of two rounds of breath here

- Feel the throat from the inside out; let it fully fill the space.

Leave a silence of two rounds of breath here

- Becoming aware of that point just between the eyebrows, let it soften and expand.

Leave a silence of two rounds of breath here

- Imagine you are lying on a sheepskin blanket.

- You are held by a fluffy, cosy bed and your whole body sinks a little deeper.

- All the muscles soften and relax.

- Your fluffy bed lies on the ground of an incredible crystal cave.

- In this large, cavernous space beautiful, see-through quartz crystals line the walls and the ceiling.

- It's a wonderful place, like a dream.

- Just take a moment to look around the cave at the magical crystals.

- This is a place of healing.

- A special place designed to realign your *chakras*.

- The crystals can change colour and channel high vibrational light to rebalance your *chakras*.

- Watch now as the clear white crystals begin to turn a gorgeous ruby red colour.

- Just tap into your root *chakra* now.

- That space just at the base of the spine.

- Each of our *chakras* is a circular vortex of energy. When they are unbalanced they can move either too fast or get sluggish and spin too slowly.

- Our root *chakra*, at the base of the spine, symbolises our basic needs, our sense of belonging. Our sense of security. Our trust. Trust in ourselves and trust in others.

- Just focus on the sensations at the bottom of your spine. What is your root *chakra* like today? Is it spinning too fast? Too slow? Or is it just right?

Leave a silence of a few rounds of breath here

- Now invite a beam of light from one of the crystals. A beam of red light to bathe your root *chakra* in a balancing light. The vibrations carried on the light will bring the *chakra* back into balance. Speeding up or slowing down until it reaches equilibrium.

- There is nothing for you to do. The light's natural qualities restore balance.

Leave a silence of a few rounds of breath here

- Watch now as the crystals change from red to orange. Notice all the different tones of orange shining in the crystals.

- Take your awareness to your sacral *chakra* now, which is in your lower abdomen, just below your navel. It is our centre of creativity, wellbeing and pleasure.

- Just watch the *chakra* for a few moments. What do you find here? Is this circle of orange energy spinning too fast, too slow or does it feel just right?

Leave a silence of a few rounds of breath here

- Invite a beam of orange light from a crystal to bathe and realign your sacral *chakra* now.

- Feel the sensations of the light pouring into your *chakra* and bringing it back into a steady balance.

- Bringing with it a sense of wellbeing.

Leave a silence of a few rounds of breath here

- Become aware of the glow of light in the cave now shifting from orange to yellow. Notice the crystals in their yellow splendour.

- Drop the internal gaze now to the solar plexus, that point just below the ribs but just above the belly button. Drop the awareness deep into the body at this point and see what you find.

- Our solar plexus deals with our power, our levels of confidence and self-worth. What do you find here? We are just observing with no judgement, just being curious about what we find.

- Draw a beam of sunny yellow light through the crystal, right into the solar plexus.

- Just notice what happens.

- Let the crystal-charged light do its work. Relax and let go.

Leave a silence of around two rounds of breath here

- Now notice as the crystal transitions from yellow to an incredible green colour.

- Drop the awareness into the heart space to locate your heart *chakra* that holds our love, our sense of self-acceptance and our healing qualities.

- Locate your heart *chakra*, your wheel of energy, and just notice, with no judgement, how it is spinning.

Leave a silence of a few rounds of breath here

- Notice the change as the green light from one of the crystals beams directly into your heart, directly into the centre of your energy wheel, and brings the spinning back into balance.

Leave a silence of around two rounds of breath here

- The colour of the crystal moves into turquoise and then into a brilliant blue. Take a moment to admire the shining blue crystals and the change of vibration it brings to the space.

- Inhabiting the space in the throat now, the centre point of the neck, your throat *chakra*. Which works with our communication. Our self-expression. Our truth.

- Take the internal gaze to the centre of the throat and just sense what is there.

Leave a silence of a few rounds of breath here

- Invite a beam of blue crystal light into the *chakra* and let go, just observing what happens.

Leave a silence of a few rounds of breath here

- Watch as the cave's crystals transition from blue through to indigo.

- Deep purple shades shine through.

- Notice the point just between the eyebrows, this is your brow *chakra*, your third eye. Your centre of intuition and awareness. Linked to your sense of purpose and direction in life. Just soften the internal gaze at this point.

Leave a silence of a few rounds of breath here

- A beam of indigo light shines, directing onto your third eye. Kinaesthetically feel the indigo light beaming into your third eye.

Leave a silence of a few rounds of breath here

- The crystals in the cave slowly begin to shift from indigo to purple now.

- Notice a point just above the top of your head. See if you can feel your crown *chakra.* Your energy vortex spinning just above the crown of your head. Let it spin and just observe it. Our crown *chakra* is our connection to the divine. The divine in us and seeing the divine in others.

Leave a silence of a few rounds of breath here

- Invite a beam of purple light to bathe the crown *chakra.* You don't need to do anything at all. Just watch and feel. Think about the connection to your divine, inner self. Open that link to the connection.

Leave a silence of a few rounds of breath here

- Watch now as the colour slowly leaves the crystals and they turn back to the clear crystals that they began as.

- Just come back to the sensation of the fluffy sheepskin rug underneath you now. See if the full weight of the body can rest more fully onto the blanket.

- Widen your internal lens to take in your body as a whole now, and just notice the little glowing coloured *chakras* aligned in your body.

- Notice that sense of profound wellbeing and balance.

Leave a silence of a few rounds of breath here

- Send an inhale up the central channel of your being. Exhale slowly to release.

- Hold those *chakras* in line and in balance, slowly coming back onto your mat.

- Notice where your body rests in the space in the room.

- Gently shake your head from side to side.

- Bring a little movement into your fingers and your toes.

- Stretch out in any way that would feel good.

- And when you are ready, open your eyes.

CHAPTER 5

Writing Your Own Guided Meditation Scripts

This chapter outlines how to create your own guided meditation scripts. All our students have different needs and it is great to personalise scripts to embrace their unique needs. It's wonderful how many different yoga classes there are today. From children's yoga, mother and baby yoga, yoga for people with cancer, all the way through to golden years yoga for older people. So this chapter is to support you in writing great guided meditation scripts that will resonate with your students.

The right headspace

Before you begin writing a script, it's beneficial to get into the right headspace, and this can be done in two ways:

- Consider who you are writing for and what their needs are. From this, jot down themes or emotions that would be helpful for the group to cultivate. It is our main aim in writing these scripts that the students have a positive experience and for them to feel better in body and mind after the meditation than they did before.

- Relax yourself. It is beneficial to the writing process to be in a similar state that the students will be in during the meditation when you are writing it. This way your students will be able to readily connect with your words and your message. You can relax by doing some yoga yourself, by going for a walk, meditating, or by doing all three! From a relaxed, calm and steady mind, the writing will flow.

Position

Consider what position you would like the students in. As discussed earlier in the book, this is generally seated or lying down, but always take into consideration modifications or props you may need. Additionally, think about how long your meditation will be. For a short meditation of around 5 minutes, it is suitable to have students seated. However, unless they are experienced yogis, this may become uncomfortable after a while. Therefore, if your meditation is a longer one, anywhere from 10 minutes, it may be best to have them lying down.

Writing the script
Relax the mind

When you begin a meditation script it is best to allow the students to mentally arrive in the space. Allow them to relax by asking them to shift their focus from the thoughts in the mind and to come back to the sensations of the body. This is done in two stages, via the breath and safe space.

Breath

The first stage of relaxing is settling the breath. This moves awareness from the mind to the breath, and also helps to regulate the breath back to a natural pattern. Some students will have been shallow breathing in their chest all day or all week without realising it, and one of the quickest ways to stimulate our parasympathetic nervous system (PNS), our destress button, is to simply lengthen the exhalation.

Begin by asking your students to take a full inhalation into the belly and then exhale slowly to release. It's best to do at least three rounds of deep breathing here. Below are a few options on how to instruct this, and you can use these, or come up with your own ideas:

- On the inhale count to four, and on the exhale count to six.

- Inhale deeply into the belly. With a sigh, exhale.

- Inhale into the belly, draw the inhale into the lungs. Exhale slowly, with a sense of letting go.

- Inhale from the head all the way down to the toes. Exhale from the toes to the crown of the head.

- Feel the breath being received into the belly. Gently release on the exhale.

- Inhale what you need into the belly. Exhale, release and let go of anything that no longer serves the body.

- Feel the stretch of the skin across the belly on the inhale, and notice the release of the belly on the exhale.

Safe space

It is at this point that you may wish to point out to the students that they are in a safe space. This can be done directly by saying something like:

- This is a safe space. A space to honour the needs of your body today.

Or, if you would prefer to say it indirectly, you could say something along the lines of:

- You are held in this space. Allow the muscles in the body to relax and drop a little more.

Or:

- Allow your mat to hold you in the space. Let the full weight of the body rest on your mat.

Body sensations

To further relax the student, they should now focus on the sensations of their bodies, again, as an anchor to focus their awareness and as an opportunity to reconnect with themselves as they go deeper into relaxation. There are endless possibilities here. Below are a few examples.

Body scan

Guide your students through a simple body scan, starting either at the head or the toes. I prefer to start at the toes, as it draws awareness to the opposite end of the body from the mind. You can invite the students to imagine a blue relaxing liquid entering the body via the tips of the toes, or any other vehicle to move the relaxing sensations around the body, for example a golden light or silver mist. The aim at this stage is not to change anything, just to be the observer, checking in with how the body feels at the present moment. So invite the student just to notice what they find with a sense of curiosity and no judgement. Remind them that if the mind wanders, that's fine, that's what it does, and with a loving breath, bring it back to your voice and where you want the focus to be.

Face

The face is a good one to focus on as it is a place where we commonly hold tension without realising it. Ask the students to notice the point between the eyebrows and to let it soften. Then draw the focus to the eyes and imagine a smile spreading across the eyes. This simple act stimulates their nervous system and they begin to relax. You could ask them to relax the jaw and release the tongue from the top of the mouth. Ask them to relax down to the root of the tongue and notice the sensations in the mouth, the teeth, the gums, and between the lips.

Body parts

One way to get students to notice and reconnect with their body parts is to imagine breathing down them. You could ask them to breathe down their entire right leg on an inhale and then exhale back up the leg. You could do this for three rounds of breath. Have a break of silence to settle the mind and breath, and then see how it feels to do this on the left leg.

Emotions

You can use the heart as a vehicle for the students to check in with their emotions in this present moment. Draw the awareness to the heart by asking the students to rest a hand on the heart. Show that it's a nurturing attention by asking them to adjust the touch so that it feels tender and light. Or if you'd rather they keep their body still, bring the focus to the heart by allowing the breath to be felt there. Then ask if they can give space to everything that the heart has been carrying this week. Ask them to give space to feelings of happiness, excitement and peace, but also ask them to give space to feelings of hurt, of sadness, or loneliness. Sometimes we don't even know what we are carrying until we shine a light on it. Then ask them to offer some attention to whatever needs it, to offer love, kindness, compassion, or anything else.

Prana

You can use the palms of the hands for the students to check in with their *prana*. This is especially helpful if you will be doing any work with energy or *mudras*. With the palms facing up, ask the students to drop the awareness into the palms of the hands and take a moment to see what they find there. See if they can begin to notice any heat or warmth coming from the palms of the hands. Then see if they can access that more subtle layer of energy or *prana* being released by the palms of the hands. Give them time just to observe what's there. Ask if they can feel the movement of energy. Does it have a colour? What's the sensation? Pause here just to give the students time to notice, and then ask if both hands feel exactly the same or whether one is releasing more than the other.

The 'peak'

The next stage is the 'peak' of the guided meditation. This is the part of the script where you can cultivate that positive feeling or emotion or release, and let go of anything negative. There are a multitude of themes or emotions you can work on here. Similarly, there are endless 'vehicles' or guided imagery you can use as the means to get your message across.

One of the most common is a journey with a starting point, like a forest, where the student begins their journey by going down a path. The middle of the journey could be them coming across an object that will give them strength or courage, for example. The end could be them carrying on the path, walking with more confidence and ease before arriving home. Some of the elements of the journey can be symbolic, like a fire symbolising courage and strength, or you can name the qualities you want to cultivate.

A setting in nature is always a good starting point as it is naturally relaxing and open to interpretation so the students can tailor their own experience. Beaches, forests, gardens or any natural landscape are all beautiful calming spaces that we can conjure up as personal pictures in our mind's eye in a moment. Try not to give too much description in the script to allow the students to connect with their own version. Ask the students what certain aspects look, feel or smell like. The more they kinaesthetically connect to the experience, the more they benefit from it.

The most important aspect is that it comes with the students' best interests at heart. Your class will determine the theme you want to work with. Of course there are many universal themes, including cultivating compassion, or a loving kindness-focused meditation. If your class is a children's yoga class you can work more on stories, which could include morals or being a good friend as a theme. If you are running a parent and baby class, it could be a destressing or nurturing theme.

It's also good to bear in mind that just because it is a guided meditation, this doesn't mean the peak has to be complex. If anything, it's better to err on the side of simplicity. You could do a whole peak about the sensations of floating on a cloud, or the presence of *prana* in our body. If we make it too complex, the mind is stimulated too much and it switches from being relaxed to being alert. Our main aim is to take our students to a deep level of relaxation and to release as many layers of tension, and bring about a relaxed but content and balanced state.

It is also important to take your time. Leave a short silence of at least a round of breath after reading each line. This is beneficial in two ways. First, it lets the student fully realise in their mind's eye the message or image you have presented. Second, it lets you read over the next line, so when you read it out loud, it flows naturally. Leave silences anywhere from 10 seconds up to a minute throughout, depending on when you see fit, so the students can fully immerse themselves in the experience.

Coming back

When you have finished the peak, gently guide the students back. This can begin with a space of silence of around a minute for the students to take in the messages, images or story of the peak. You can guide them back in a few stages. First, ask them to take a deep breath into their belly. Then invite them to notice a physical sensation. This will bring them back into their bodies and into the room. You could ask them to notice:

- The back of their head resting on the mat, or

- The outer edge of their body and the touch of the atmosphere on the skin, or

- Sensations in the soles of their feet.

Next bring them round a little more, by bringing a little movement into the body. You may ask them to:

- Gently shake their head from side to side.

- Bring a little movement back into their fingers and toes.

- Stretch out or reach out in any way that would feel good.

- Come into any pose they need to, to complete their practice, for example, a happy baby or *apanasana* or a twist.

After the students have finished stretching, ask them to roll over onto their right-hand side; they can rest their head on the inside of the right arm. And when they are ready, they can come up to sit.

Settle them back into *sukhasana*. Take one more full round of breath into the belly. This completes their gentle transition back into the room, so when they are ready, ask them to open their eyes.

Things to avoid

Our main aim is to keep the students very relaxed. Therefore we don't want to present them with any imagery, story or thought that might conjure up fear or any other negative feeling. The student will, of course, interpret the meditation in their own way, we have no control over that; but just be mindful to keep all material in a very safe space. Consider the aspects below before writing.

Setting

Try not to use any setting that may be viewed as claustrophobic, scary or uncomfortable. For example, images of a cave might frighten some. Similarly, a city may feel too busy for a relaxing meditation. Keeping the description of a setting vague is helpful as the students can imagine their own peaceful setting, for example, 'an open field' or 'a beach'.

Religion

Try to avoid all religious terminology or imagery as you don't know the religious beliefs or lack of beliefs of your students. Although yoga has firm roots in Hinduism, yoga itself is generally viewed as a non-religious concept.

Imagery

Be mindful of the imagery you present and if it has any other meanings. For example, a red poppy could be viewed as a beautiful flower, but to many it will represent the fallen soldiers of the First World War.

Glossary

anjali – to offer/to salute.

apanasana – a yoga pose where the student is lying on their back with their knees drawn into the chest.

asana – a yoga pose.

chakra – a spinning energy vortex in the body; we have seven of them.

chin – consciousnesses.

hasta – hand.

hasta mudra – hand gesture.

Hathayogapradipika – 15th-century Sanskrit manual on Hatha Yoga.

hridaya – heart.

Iyengar – a prominent yoga teacher who developed a style of yoga named after himself.

Kali – named after the fearsome goddess Durga.

Kularnava Tantra – an ancient text on the tantra tradition.

manas – mind.

mantra – a sacred sound, syllable, word or group of words.

mudra – gesture/seal.

nadis – invisible channels around the body that carry *prana*.

prana – life force.

pranayama – breath/breath control/extension of *prana*.

Sanskrit – language of ancient India dating back around 3500 years.

shavasana – corpse pose.

sukhasana – easy sitting pose.

ujjayi – a breathing technique performed in yoga.

vishuddha – throat *chakra*.

yogi – a practitioner of yoga.

yoni – womb/source.

References

Albertson, E.R., Neff, K.D. and Dill-Shackleford, K.E. (2014) 'Self-compassion and body dissatisfaction in women: A randomised controlled trial of a brief meditation intervention.' *Mindfulness 6*, 444–454. doi:10.1007/s12671-014-0277-3

Elomaa, M.M., de Williams, A.C. and Kalso, E.A. (2009) 'Attention management as a treatment for chronic pain.' *European Journal of Pain 13*, 1062–1067. doi:10.1016/j.ejpain.2008.12.002

Eremin, O., Walker, M.B., Simpson, E., Heys, S.D., Ah-See, A.K., Hutcheon, A.W., *et al.* (2009) 'Immuno-modulatory effects of relaxation training and guided imagery in women with locally advanced breast cancer undergoing multimodality therapy: A randomised controlled trial.' *Breast 18*, 1, 17–25. doi:10.1016/j.breast.2008.09.002

Fernros, L., Furhoff, A.-K. and Wandell, P.E. (2008) 'Improving quality of life using compound mind-body therapies: Evaluation of a course intervention with body movement and breath therapy, guided imagery, chakra experiencing and mindfulness meditation.' *Quality of Life Research 17*, 367–376. doi:10.1007/s11136-008-9321-x

Gard, T., Noggle, J.J., Park, C.L., Vago, D.R. and Wilson, A. (2014) 'Potential self-regulatory mechanisms of yoga for psychological health.' *Frontiers in Human Neuroscience 8*, 770. doi:10.3389/fnhum.2014.00770

Goyal, M., Singh, S., Sibinga, E.M.S., Gould, N.F., Rowland-Seymour, A., Sharma, R., *et al.* (2014) 'Meditation programs for psychological stress and well-being.' *JAMA Internal Medicine 174*, 3, 357–368. doi:10.1001/jamainternmed.2013.13018

Jain, S., McMahon, G.F., Hasen, P., Kozub, M.P., Porter, V., King, R. and Guarneri, E.M. (2012) 'Healing touch with guided imagery for PTSD in returning active duty.' *Military Medicine 177*, 9, 1015–1021.

Lim, D., Condon, P. and DeSteno, D. (2014) 'Mindfulness and compassion: An examination of mechanism and scalability.' *PLOS One*, 17 February. doi:10.1371/journal.pone.0118221

Melville, G., Chang, D., Colagiuri, B., Marshall, P. and Cheema, B. (2012) 'Fifteen minutes of yoga postures or guided meditation in the office can elicit psychological and physiological relaxation.' *International Research Congress on Integrative Medicine and Health.*

Sarang, P.S. and Telles, S. (2006) 'Oxygen consumption and respiration during and after two yoga relaxation techniques.' *Applied Psychophysiology and Biofeedback 31*, 2, 143–153.

Saraswati, S.S. (1969) *Asana Pranayama Mudra Bandha.* Munger, Bihar, India: Yoga Publications Trust, p.421.

Saraswati, S.S. (1976) 'The Art of Relaxation.' In S.S. Saraswati, *Yoga Nidra*. Munger, Bihar, India: Yoga Publications Trust, p.14.

Schneiderman, N., Ironson, G. and Siegle, S.D. (2005) 'Stress and health: Psychological, behavioural, and biological determinants.' *Annual Review of Clinical Psychology 1*, 607–628. doi:10.1146/annurev.clinpsy.1.102803.144141

Shapiro, A.K. (1959) 'The placebo effect in the history of medical treatment.' *American Journal of Psychiatry 116*, 4, 298–304.

Taimni, I.K. (1972) *The Science of Yoga: The Yoga-Sutras of Patanjali in Sanskrit*. Adyar, Chennai, India: The Theosophical Publishing House.

Telles, S., Reddy, S.K. and Nagendra, H.R. (2000) 'Oxygen consumption and respiration following two yoga relaxation techniques.' *Applied Psychophysiology and Biofeedback 25*, 4, 221–227.

Tosevski, D.L., Lecic, D., *et al.* (2006) 'Stressful life events and physical health.' *Current Opinion in Psychology 19*, 2, 184–189.

Vyas, A., Mitra, R., Rao, B.S.S. and Chattarji, S. (2002) 'Chronic stress induces contrasting patterns of dendritic remodeling in hippocampal and amygdaloid neurons.' *Journal of Neuroscience 22*, 15, 6810–6818. doi.org/10.1523/JNEUROSCI.22-15-06810.2002

Wells, J. (2010) 'Transpersonal Awareness, Mindfulness Meditation, and Guided Imagery: A Qualitative Study Using Concise Narrative Vignettes.' Dissertation Abstracts International: Section B. Sciences and Engineering, p.70.

Index